The
Savvy Woman's Guide
to
Testosterone

How to Revitalize Your
Sexuality, Strength and Stamina

D1241943

by Elizabeth Lee Vliet, M.D.

The Savvy Woman's Guide to Testosterone
by Elizabeth Lee Vliet, M.D.
Copyright © 2005 Elizabeth Lee Vliet, M.D.

Published by:
HER Place Press
PO Box 64507
Tucson AZ 85728-4507
www.herplace.com

Disclaimer:
The ideas and suggestions in this book are based on the clinical experience and medical training of the author and scientific articles available. Every attempt has been made to present current and accurate information as of the time of publication. The suggestions in this book are definitely *not* meant to be a substitute for careful medical evaluation and treatment by a qualified, licensed health professional. Each women's health needs, risks, and goals are different and should be developed with medical supervision for personalized advice, answers to specific medical questions, and individual recommendations. The author and publisher specifically do not recommend starting any new treatment, changing any medication you may be taking, or using over-the-counter hormone preparations without consulting your personal physician. This book is intended for educational purposes only, and the use of the information is entirely at the reader's discretion. The author and publisher cannot be responsible for any adverse reactions arising directly or indirectly from the suggestions in this material, and specifically disclaim any liability from the use of this book.

All of the patient vignettes described in the book are actual patients from the author's medical practice and have not been created just for this book. Names, and if necessary, identifying details, have been changed to preserve patient confidentiality but these changes did not alter the actual clinical information, lab results, patient comments, or treatment presented.

Cover Design: Kitty Werner, RSBPress and New West Agency
Book Design: Kitty Werner, RSBPress
Production and Prepress: Kitty Werner, RSBPress
Printed by Central Plains Book Manufacturing, Winfield KS
                   Printed on New Life Opaque 100% recycled paper

ISBN 1-933213-00-0
Library of Congress Control Number:
Printed and bound in the United States of America
0 9 8 7 6 5 4 3 2 1

The Savvy Woman's Mantra

"Nothing is obvious
to the uninformed."
—Salada tea bag tag

DEDICATION

To my patients…and readers…whose stories and struggles have inspired me to strive to be inquisitive, keep an open mind, and learn more…

To the Sexual Consultation team at Johns Hopkins during my residency, who taught me so much.

To Gordon, Kitty, and Kathy—whose hard work and support made it possible for me to meet the challenges and deadlines of writing another book while still seeing patients.

To the women who have been told, "it's all in your head," I hope this will show you how important hormones really are for women's bodies, especially testosterone!

To God who guides it all.

Author's Note

I have specialized in evaluating and treating hormone-related problems for over twenty years. I have treated thousands of women. I have seen firsthand the profound effects of low testosterone for women: the loss of sex drive and desire, the loss of ability to respond sexually or to have a normal orgasm, the bone-tired feelings, the loss of muscle strength, the loss of stamina, and most of all the loss of that spark we call zest, vitality or joie d'vivre. I have also seen and experienced the remarkable renewal in all these dimensions when healthy levels of testosterone are restored.

I know what you are going through. More than just a physician treating women, I am also a woman who has been there with you on this "hormone journey." I had a surgical menopause in my early forties. I know firsthand what the impact can be. And, I know what good hormone balance can accomplish.

My goal with this book is to overcome stigma and negative myths about testosterone for women, and teach you how to gauge benefits versus risks. You can use this book to help you sort through the maze of conflicting information and work more effectively with your own physician to find the best treatment approaches for your individual health goals. This book will help you get the most benefit from the revolutionary testosterone options available today.

The Savvy Woman's Guide to Testosterone is here to give you answers to all these issues with cutting edge medical information. I will help you understand the intricacies of proper hormone balance, benefits, safety, testing methods, optimal dosing, products, and route of delivery, and teach you practical approaches to discuss treatment options with your physicians. I will share with you my experience in helping women find the right doses, and avoid unwanted side effects of too much testosterone.

And, just as crucial as what to do to raise testosterone, I will also explain what you need to know to avoid getting overdosed with excess testosterone. I see this all too often with today's unregulated compounded, high dose creams and gels, pellets or implants. I will share with you stories from my patients, women who wanted their stories told to help prevent other women from suffering either from the loss of testosterone or from being given too much testosterone.

How much is good for you?

Too much testosterone is just as bad as too little.

Testosterone is crucial to women's health as well as men's Let's explore all that this remarkable hormone does!

Elizabeth Lee Vliet, M.D.

Tucson, AZ

February 9, 2005

Contents

Introduction.. 15

Chapter 1—The Missing Link **23**
Women's Voices, Women's Stories.................................... 24
Overview of Testosterone's Importance 29

Chapter 2—Testosterone and Androgens in Women:
What They Are and What They Do **33**
The Menstrual Cycle and Testosterone 40
Natural Menopause 46
Surgical Menopause... 46
Women and Androgen Insufficiency Syndrome (AIS)............. 48
What Causes Low Androgens, especially
    Testosterone, in Women?.. 51
Case Study 54

Chapter 3—Testosterone and Women's Sexuality **59**
It's NOT All in Your Head 60
Myths and Stereotypes of Women's Sexuality 61
Do women deserve any less? 65
Women's Sexual Response: Just What is "Normal"....... 71
Changes As We Age.. 74
Androgens as Sexual "Activators" 77
It Takes to Two to Tango... 79
Understanding A Woman's Sexual Response 81
Varieties of Women's Sexual Dysfunction 84
Restoring Your Sexual Vitality... 89

Chapter 4—Testosterone Effects Throughout
The Body.. **91**
Testosterone and Brain Effects 97
Testosterone Effects on Sleep 99
Testosterone and Hair, Skin and Eyes............................ 100
More Hormone Effects on Hair... 102
Testosterone and Estradiol Effects on
    Vulvar, Vaginal, and Urinary Problems....................... 103
Hormone Decline and Vulvar/Vestibular Pain 105
Hormone Decline and Urinary Incontinence................ 107
Summary 110

Chapter 5—Dispelling the Myths and
Misunderstandings **111**
Let's Set the Record Straight 113

Behind the Headlines 121
Critical Points Overlooked in the News.......................... 126
Take Home Messages 127
Dealing with Your Insurance Plan 128
Case Study: Patti's Story... 128
Summary: Be in Charge—Speak UP! 130

**Chapter 6—Old Approaches to Testosterone
Therapy...131**
Myths About "Male Hormones" for Women.................... 136
Compounded Testosterone Products 138
Toxic Testosterone Cream 140
Androgen Overload.. 142
Too Much Testosterone 146
Problems with Combo Products 149
Cautions 151

Chapter 7—DHEA: Promises and Pitfalls 153
What is DHEA and Where Is It Made? 157
DHEA Patterns Through Our Life Cycle 159
DHEA: Concerns and Cautions for Women.................... 160
Promises and Potential for the Future 163
DHEA and Cognitive Function 163
DHEA and Mood.. 164
DHEA and Bone 165
DHEA and Immune Function 165
DHEA and Sex Drive 166
DHEA and Fertility Treatment 167
DHEA in Addison's Disease and Hypopituitarism 167
Replacing DHEA in Addison's Disease............................ 168

**Chapter 8—The Testosterone Revolution for Women:
Restoring Your Sexuality, Energy and Vitality 173**
Bioidentical Testosterone 173
Pills, Potions, Lotions, or Shots? 174
Oral Tablets and Capsules 177
Creams and Patches.. 180
Gels and Troches.. 181
Injectables 181
Pellets and Implants 182
Topical preparations for the vagina and vulva........... 183
New Products in the Pipeline. 184
Dosing Issues 185
Update on Testosterone and Breast Cancer Risk 187

Let's explore what we know at this time 188
Finding What's Right for You: Tracking Your Responses 193

Chapter 9—Testosterone ACTION Plan: Restoring Your Hormone Balance for Zest, Vitality …and Feeling Sexy Again! 195
What Should Be Measured? 196
What about Saliva and Urine Hormone Tests? 197
What Other Tests Should Be Done? 199
Your Hormone Tests and What They Mean 199
Your Bone Markers and Other Tests 205
Finding "Optimal" Levels verses "Normal"
   Reference Ranges 207
Benefits of Comprehensive Hormone Testing 207
Beyond the Blood Tests: Putting It All Together 209
Effects of progesterone/progestins on testosterone 211
In Summary 215
Chart: Your Hormone Power Life Plan®
Dr. Vliet's STARTING STEPS: 216

Chapter 10—Become the Savvy, New You! Putting it All Together 219
Sensate Focus 221
Lifestyle Thieves of Sexual Vitality 224
Get Going and Move That Body! 226
Healthy Eating For Energy and Vitality…
   and Feeling Sexier 228
Doctor, I Need To Talk! 230
It's A New World Out There 233
It's Called Quality of Life 234
And in Conclusion… 241

Appendix I—Glossary of Medical Terms 243
I. List of Medical Acronyms Used in This Book 243
II. Medical Terms Defined 244

Appendix II—Bibliography and Resources 263
I. MEDICAL BIBLIOGRAPHY 263
II. Groups and Organizations 276
Sources For Natural Hormones 277
General Comments about Compounded Hormones 278
Compounded Hormones vs. FDA-Approved Hormones 279

To Contact Dr. Vliet 280

Acknowledgments

My deepest thanks and appreciation to all who have made this book possible—especially the dedicated researchers and clinicians worldwide who have led the way in providing the science to show how important testosterone is for women's bodies. In particular, pioneers such as Drs. Robert Greenblatt, Morrie Gelfand, Barbara Sherwin, Philip Sarrel, Peter Casson, and Professor A.R. Genazzani, have been instrumental in researching the role of androgens in cognitive, mood and sexual function in women, and in developing appropriate androgen therapies for women. I have learned much from your work that has enabled me to help others.

I am grateful for the trust placed in me by my patients, many of whom have had long struggles trying to find answers and help for puzzling hormone-related problems. You have honored me by sharing your experiences and had the confidence to allow me to guide you on the journey to better health. We are students and teachers of one another in this hormone journey as women, which can certainly be both "marvelous *and* maddening." Your insights and observations have taught me much that goes beyond the textbooks of medicine. This book becomes part of your legacy too, as I pass on your experiences so that they can touch others and help women know the truth of their own body experiences.

I also appreciate those of you who are not patients, but have read my books, found them helpful to you in your own health journey and enabled you to use the information to work with your own physicians. Thank you for letting me know that my books have made a difference and served to extend my reach beyond the four walls of my patient office.

As one reader recently wrote: "*I am a 39-year-old who recently found out I have osteoporosis. It's amazed me that an*

Endo, Gyn and Neuro all had no clue that my bones were affected by low androgens. I would never have known as much as I know without your books, so I thank you from the bottom of my heart. I have been a computer guru since the 80s and it's rare that I can find more info from books than from searching online, but that's definitely the case with your books. Thanks for your technical take, details, and recognizing that androgen deficiency really exists." Thank you for sharing your story…it makes the hard work of writing books all worthwhile!

My deepest gratitude to my husband, Gordon Vliet, who as always, has been the "the wind beneath my wings," and once again has gone through all the pressures and joys of working with me on another book, as well as helping to run the office and care for our patients. You are, and have always been, the love of my life, and the best support and encouragement I could possibly have.

Kudos to Kitty Werner, designer and typesetter par excellence, whose boundless enthusiasm for this book and always positive, "can-do" attitude helped to get this project off the ground. Her design ideas and meticulous craftsmanship in production I feel has led to a book that is both pleasing to the eye, and easy to read and use. I am grateful for her wisdom, expertise, and guidance… and creativity for the title! She's a *real* savvy woman!

Much appreciation again to Kathy Kresnik, who in the midst of many other responsibilities and stresses with her three boys and their own surging androgens, once again labored long hours to help with the research, writing, *rewriting,* reading and re-reading tasks to bring this book into being. She has a special understanding of the role of stress in sapping a busy mother's energy!

Special thanks to Berit Jones, Claudia Sawyer, Sherry Grimm and Polly Leigh. Your positive attitude, dedication, and commitment to support my work, and to be a caring presence for our patients, have been invaluable. All of you have blossomed in your roles in caring for our patients and overseeing daily office operations to keep our clinical offices responsive to the needs of our patients while I take the time and energy to focus on researching and writing. Thank you for your support and encouragement.

Thanks also to Tom Wadkins, business and financial overseer, computer whiz, and operations manager who has brought our operations into the 21st century in so many ways, and made my job easier. Thanks for always willingly been available to solve my technical challenges and glitches to keep the projects moving ahead. My appreciation to my business advisors, David Cohen, C.P.A., and Tony Rickert—who guide me through the complexities of accounting and legal aspects of running the medical practices.

Thanks to Becky Simpson of New West Agency, who was invaluable with her design input for the cover. And thanks to Lynne O'Hara and her team at Chelsea Green Publishing, and Melody Morris and the team at Central Plains Manufacturing, for all their work in production, printing, distribution and sales to help get this important message out to more women.

Thanks to the friends, colleagues, and patients who reviewed the early stages of the manuscript and gave me important guidance to make this book even better. The eagle eyes of Virginia Davis and Margaret Jordan, both grammatical purists, once again provided invaluable editing help. Two busy professional women, LFH and MB, were especially helpful with suggestions to refine this book to make it helpful to readers, yet keep the scientific grounding that women need to understand complex issues. All of my reader-editor "team" know firsthand the trial and tribulations of the "hormonal challenges" woman face, and how important this information is to women of all ages. All are inspiring examples that woman of all ages can learn more about their bodies, master complex material and use it to take the necessary steps to feel better.

I thank the many health professionals—physicians, nurse practitioners, registered nurses, psychologists, physical therapists and others—have read my books, thought they made sense and were scientifically "sound" to the point that they have sent patients, or have come themselves, for hormone evaluations. I thank you for your trust in my knowledge and approaches, and I thank you for the validation that your comments have given me. You become the additional messengers taking this crucial message back to your communities and to the women whose lives you touch in your professional work.

Together, we all make a difference, and make positive changes toward a truly *woman-centered* healthcare model for the future that will incorporate our unique hormone makeup as a fundamental part of our being that needs to be included in all our health assessments and treatment planning.

Elizabeth Lee Vliet, M.D.

Tucson, Arizona

February 9, 2005

Introduction

So, you are approaching another birthday, closer and closer to the next "big" one. One of those years ending in a zero.

Your *body* is changing. Hard not to notice. Flabby arms, expanding waist, cellulite thighs, tummy fat. You may have tried weight training, fitness walks, and memberships at fitness centers. But, none of that seems to do much good to keep your body shapely and toned.

Your *mind* may be subtly changing, too. Maybe you feel like your energy level and mental sharpness aren't what they used to be. Maybe you feel dull and blah more of the time. You exercise and eat right and still feel mentally and physically exhausted, like you've hit a brick wall. What's going on?

Maybe you don't have your sexual spark anymore. Maybe it scares you that you don't even miss it. Has sex become something you and your friends just joke about? After a day at the office, a long commute home, the carpool to pick up kids, fixing a quick dinner, doing the dishes and two loads of laundry, helping the kids with homework…do you have the time or energy for sex? Has sex become just another chore? When you do make love do you feel the same intensity or pleasure you once had enjoyed?

That's what this book is all about—helping you find the answers to revitalize your sex drive, get back that sexy feeling again, along with that missing energy, strength, and stamina.

It's no joke

Has sex become something you and your friends just joke about?

Now, you can do something about it.

Kelly's Story

Kelly, age 39, was worried as her birthday approached. It wasn't the number of years, it was her body. Subtle, but noticeable, changes. She thought, *"I still look good, at least in clothes."* Her once athletic and muscular arms now reminded her of her mother's flabby ones. Even weight training no longer did much good to keep her arms shapely and toned. After her hysterectomy at age 37 when both ovaries were removed, her energy level and sharp, clear thinking never fully returned. She exercised, took her estrogen and was thankful she didn't suffer the usual hot flashes and other consequences of hysterectomy. But still, something was missing.

Ain't it the truth!

All she wanted was seven hours of uninterrupted sleep...and here he is, looking at her with a glint in his eye.

Sex. Sex was what was missing. She was caught up being a busy mom, running kids around town, keeping up the house, and oh yeah, working part-time. She was exhausted most of the time. She didn't have the energy for sex much anymore. The disturbing part was she didn't really miss it. Sex had become just another item on her "have to do" list.

But underneath it all, what really alarmed her was that she didn't even desire sex. *"This isn't like me,"* she thought. *"Sex used to be fun, a big part of our time together. I loved it. What's wrong with me?"* Now, when she and her husband did make love, she had a harder time getting aroused, and didn't feel the same pleasure she once had enjoyed. Orgasm? That now felt like it was gone before she realized it had happened. Her husband was beginning to notice it, too. All she wanted was seven hours of uninterrupted sleep...and here he is looking at her with a glint in his eye. Was this how it was to be? Should she just accept this new way of feeling, or try to find some way to "fix it?"

Kelly felt she was too young to just give up on sex...yet, what could she do? She increased her exercise in hopes this would increase her energy levels and interest in sex, too. But her muscles still felt weak and flabby. She had been an athlete in high school and college and had toned, strong muscles then. She knew what training and exercise could do to build muscles, but now this wasn't happening. Her body just didn't respond to exercise the way it used to. She was frustrated, worried, and a little scared. She really was much too young to feel such a loss of strength. She made an effort to eat right and take vitamins, and still she couldn't lose that stubborn fifteen pounds…much of it now around her waist and middle body, a marked change for someone used to having a trim figure.

Heads Up:

When it comes to your hormones, your doctor may need an education.

She knew something was wrong, so she asked her doctor to check her hormones. He just told her that wasn't necessary, and told her she needed to rent a seductive movie and buy some sexy lingerie. Kelly felt dismissed and even ashamed after this visit, like it was somehow her fault she wasn't much interested in sex anymore.

She knew there was a vibrant woman still inside her, full of life…but where? How to get her back? It was overwhelming. She lacked the motivation to even try and find her. She felt like someone had pulled the plug not only on her sex drive but on her "get-up-and go." "*It has been two years since my hysterectomy and ovaries were removed,*" she thought, "*surely I should have recovered by now…or is this as good as it gets?*" The unanswered questions nagged and haunted her.

"*What happened to my sex drive?*"

"*What happened to my energy?*"

"*Why am I so bone-tired all the time?*"

"*What happened to my muscle tone—I feel like mush.*"

Is This You?

There are millions of you having the problems Kelly faced. Best estimates? Tens of millions of women suffering in silence. Agonizing inwardly over lost sex drive. Befuddled by loss of energy and stamina. Indeed, studies have found that when asking doctors about hormone problems, women report fatigue second only to loss of libido. Many times they have to will themselves to get through each day. They feel their bodies have become strangers. Often they are too embarrassed to admit it. I know—they tell me when I see them for a consultation, and say things like "I have never told anyone all this before, I was too ashamed. I thought I was the only one having these problems."

Doctors aren't much help when women do ask for solutions. Even well-meaning doctors say things like, "Just take a vacation, you're too stressed." Or, "You're getting older, that's what happens." Or, "Just rent a sexy movie." Or, "Get a vibrator." Or, "Buy a sexy nighty." Or, "You should see a sex therapist." Or, "You are depressed. Take Prozac."

Heads Up!

There can be *hormone* causes of fatigue and low sex drive...

It's not "just stress."

Almost never do doctors suggest there may be physical causes of low sex drive and fatigue.

Almost never do doctors check a woman's testosterone level, even though this would be routine for men with low libido.

All of the talk therapy, sex counseling, pretty lingerie, and adult toys won't bring your sexy self back if your hormones aren't right. Your ovarian hormones are your metabolic fuel to energize the body and mind. Especially testosterone, the overlooked "woman's" hormone.

Why Testosterone?

Testosterone is a crucial part of our health picture. Most of the time, however, women don't know that testosterone, with a foundation of optimal estradiol, is critical for our sexual desire, arousal, and orgasm. Or, that testosterone affects every cell and tissue in our bodies. Its effects can be for good or ill, depending on its balance with our core female hormones, estradiol and progesterone, and "other" male hormones like DHEA.

Medical science has known about the potential benefits of testosterone for women for over fifty years. Yet five decades of basic research, clinical studies and published articles in well-respected medical journals have been mostly ignored by physicians treating women.

Ask a doctor today about testosterone for women, and you will find that most physicians are clueless about the crucial roles this powerful hormone plays in women's health. Even with hundreds of medical articles describing the benefits of testosterone, very few physicians add testosterone for women when considering hormone therapy.

Failure to restore testosterone for women—especially for those who have lost their ovaries to surgery or effects of disease—leads to untold suffering.

Testosterone for women cannot be ignored any longer. You need the facts. You need to know how to take action. That's what this book is about.

Change Starts Here—

We can change the system, but it starts with us, and one doctor at a time.

The Revolution in Women's Health Care

The Savvy Woman's Guide to Testosterone is part of a revolution in women's health. We must learn to take charge of our own health care options so we will have optimal zest and vitality as we age.

Those of us in the "baby boomer" generation are at the forefront of this revolution. Indeed, we have already revolutionized everything about our lives—our occupations, when and how we work, participation in sports, controlling our reproductive life, changing the face and experience of childbirth, creating new approaches to raising children, leading community and political agendas, challenging old myths about how we age, and dictating how we want to die.

Baby boomers have already revolutionized approaches to menopause. Clearly, we are not going "quietly into the night" as we pass into the next phase of our lives! We want and deserve answers and options to help us feel energetic, healthy—and sexy—as we age. New testosterone therapy options for women are becoming available, and older ones already in use are coming more into our awareness.

Join us!

Now it is *our* turn.

It's time for testosterone to revolutionize our approaches to women's sexual response, much as Viagra revolutionized the treatment of erection problems in men. Viagra removed the stigma of sexual dysfunction for men, removed the shaming label of "psychogenic impotence," and helped it become socially acceptable to talk about the problem.

Time for Us

Women's loss of sexual desire, and all the additional health problems that go with loss of testosterone, have been woefully overlooked by the medical profession and labeled a psychological problem. Now women have a chance to learn more about the crucial role hormones play in our sexual desire, strength and stamina.

I want to remove the stigma of testosterone for women, and teach you about the powers of this remarkable woman's hormone so that you are empowered with reliable information to talk with your health professionals about your needs.

But contrary to media hype, testosterone is not just the new "Viagra" for women. It does not work the way Viagra does in men to promote erection. Testosterone is involved in many more systems and functions in our bodies than the limited pathways affected by Viagra. Women's sexual problems and loss of desire are more complicated than simply "fixing the plumbing" for erection in men.

Women's sexual response is affected by many factors, and is much less understood by most of the medical profession.

I will explain other common causes of low libido that can occur even in young women, such as various medications, birth control pills, medical illnesses, dietary additives, life and relationship stresses and others. I will also explain the other significant symptoms of low testosterone: fatigue, depressed mood, muscle aches, loss of muscle strength and a diminished sense of well being.

Women often know intuitively when something is amiss. We need to know reliable ways to get tested to find out what it is. We need reputable information so that we can make our individual informed choices about what steps we want to take to feel better. We need safe and effective treatments to restore testosterone to its healthy balance for our bodies to function well.

The Savvy Woman's Guide to Testosterone is here to give you answers to all these issues with cutting edge medical information. I will help you understand the intricacies of proper hormone balance, benefits, safety, testing methods, optimal dosing, products, and route of delivery, and teach you practical approaches to discuss treatment options with your physicians. I will share with you my experience in helping women find the right doses, and avoid unwanted side effects of too much testosterone.

Warning:

If you don't ask the questions, your doctor may not.

And, just as crucial as what to do to raise testosterone, I will also explain what you need to know to avoid getting overdosed with excess testosterone. I see this all too often with today's unregulated compounded, high dose creams and gels, pellets or implants. I will share with you stories from my patients, women who wanted their stories told to help prevent other women from suffering either from the loss of testosterone or from being given too much testosterone.

As one of my patients so eloquently described after having healthy levels of testosterone restored:

"I feel really good! I think the addition of the testosterone was just what was needed. The muscle aches, the fatigue, my skin and losing my hair, the

crying—every single thing has gotten better. It was like a miracle! And those bladder problems I had before are completely gone now. I had terrible migraines for 20 years, I knew it was always right before my period, but now I haven't had any for a long time. That is a huge improvement for me. When I first came to you, I felt good on the estrogen. When you got that stabilized and then added the testosterone, I am really back to my old self again... and even better now!"

Testosterone is a powerful hormone. Don't live the second half of your life without it!

A Note:

Note if you don't understand a term used in the text, check the glossary and appendix for explanation.

Medical explanations and units of measure are also explained at the beginning of Appendix I.

Chapter 1

The Missing Link

Did you know that there are several ovarian hormones? Estrogen, progesterone, DHEA, and testosterone. You have heard about estrogen, over and over. Perhaps you've heard a lot about progesterone as well. You see all the ads for DHEA over the counter.

But... *Testosterone?* That's the *male* hormone isn't it? The one that makes you grow a mustache? The one that causes your voice to get deep? The one that causes liver damage?

How often have you read or heard such horror stories about testosterone? These are all old myths, based on synthetic hormones in doses designed for *men*, not for women.

Women's **ovaries** actually make *more* testosterone than estrogen during all of our reproductive lives.

I'll bet that surprises you. Most women don't know this, and neither do most doctors. No wonder testosterone has been the overlooked hormone for women.

Another little known and equally alarming fact is that as our ovary hormone production falls after menopause, we lose about *half* of our normal androgens, which includes testosterone. This loss is in addition to losing about 80% or more of our estradiol, our primary active estrogen before menopause.

Try asking a man to live the last third of his life with only half his testosterone and see what he has to say.

Women need testosterone, too. It is the hormone that

FACT:

Women make more testosterone than estrogen for *all* of our reproductive lives.

activates the sexual circuits in the brain to promote healthy sexual desire and response for both women and men. It also has a lot of other positive effects on women's bodies: it helps build healthy strong muscles, helps to build bone and prevent osteoporosis; it improves our mood and psychological well-being, to name a few of its important functions.

So now that I have your attention, let's explore some important information about testosterone for women.

Wisdom:

Before you accept a diagnosis of "it's all in your head," have your hormone levels checked.

All of them!

I find that most women have heard all the negatives, but know very little about the many beneficial roles testosterone plays in a woman's body.

In fact, in a 1993 Gallup poll of American women conducted for the North American Menopause Society, only 5% of the women polled knew that their bodies make "androgen" or that androgen levels fall after menopause.

While menopause education has come a long way in the last twelve years, there is still very limited awareness of the importance of testosterone for women.

Kelly, whom you met in the Introduction, is one of hundreds of women I have evaluated who thought her sex drive and energy level had disappeared permanently. Listen to the voices of other women I have evaluated and treated for hormone problems.

Women's Voices, Women's Stories

Kitty G—What sex drive?

"Kitty G" was a 53-year-old married woman whose periods stopped about a year-and-a-half before I saw her. She eloquently described how much she had changed since becoming menopausal:

> "I feel lethargic, I have no energy, I feel like I hit a wall everyday by 4 PM and I have had it for the day when that happens. If I sit down I'll fall asleep. And I have lots of achiness, like I have been hit by

a truck. I have hot flashes, chills, I can't sleep and my memory is shot. I don't feel like myself. I feel flat emotionally and very blah.

I love my husband and always used to really enjoy sex, but now I feel like I am dead inside, I don't have any interest in sex, and almost feel like I don't want to be touched anymore. I mentioned all this to my Gynecologist and she just gave me an antidepressant and wouldn't check my hormone levels. That made my libido totally disappear, and when I took that, I couldn't even have an orgasm at all. I don't feel depressed, just numb and flat...so I stopped the antidepressant.

I really feel it has to be something hormonal because I didn't have all these problems until my periods stopped. Along with everything else, I have been gaining weight even though I exercise four days a week, and I have these awful palpitations and pounding heart beat that make me feel like my heart is coming out of my chest. I really want some help to feel better and get my old self back."

Both her estradiol and testosterone levels were quite low, so I wasn't surprised that she felt so miserable, or that she had so many problems with her sexual response. I started her on a compounded bioidentical micronized testosterone 1 mg tablet every morning.

Since she still had her uterus and would need the progestin as well as estrogen, I suggested using Nuvaring, a vaginal ring combination of ethinyl estradiol and progestin, that could be changed once every three weeks. She liked the convenience of this approach. Six months later, Kitty reported:

"I feel so much better, I really feel great now, especially compared to what I used to feel like before I started the hormones. They have definitely made a big difference. My energy is better, I sleep better, my mood is better now. I don't have any more hot flashes

Attention!

Losing your sex drive is *not* normal.

Neither is exhaustion, irritability, lack of energy and/or lousy moods.

like I did and the pain in my joints is so much better, too. My fibromyalgia is also a lot better now and I was surprised at how much that has improved, too. I didn't think that had anything to do with hormones, but I see how much difference it made in this pain to get my hormones balanced. I am really pleased that my libido has come back! My orgasms are more intense, and sex doesn't hurt like it did when I was so dry before. My husband is really happy that I am feeling so much better—he said I was now like the woman he married."

Attention:

Getting fatter is telling you something: your hormones may be out of balance!

Now that her testosterone and estradiol were in the optimal ranges, she had the energy to exercise again, and had started doing a circuit strength training program three times a week and a Pilates class two days a week in addition to her daily brisk morning walks.

With her testosterone level now in the optimal range for women and not too high, she did not have any negative side effects as she feared might happen. She was a little worried that she had gained about four pounds on her hormones, although she noticed that her clothes were fitting much better now.

I explained that when women take hormones, and are involved with strength training exercise, they are building muscle and bone, not fat. Muscle and bone weigh about *six times* more than fat tissue, so her increase in pounds meant that with her testosterone and estradiol restored to healthy levels, her muscles could now respond to her exercise. The loss of inches made her clothes fit better and meant she had actually lost some excess body *fat*. The loss of fat did not show on her scale because exercise had increased her heavier muscle mass. Her blood pressure also went down, another benefit of improved hormone balance. Her internist was pleased and told her she could now reduce her blood pressure medicine.

Overall, Kitty was thrilled with how much better she felt. I saw her not long ago for a one-year follow-up, and she continued to be extremely pleased with the improvements in her health, energy and revitalized sex drive. She said, *"I feel so good now, I am not about to give up my hormones any time soon!"*

Susie—early menopause

Susie, a 47-year-old married homemaker, who had been started on Prempro (horse-derived conjugated estrogens with a potent synthetic progestin) about two years earlier when she went into an early menopause. She came for a consult because:

> *"I am tired of feeling so awful. I can't sleep, I have constant hot flashes, I don't have any energy at all and I just drag myself through the day. My husband is about ready to divorce me because I just don't have any interest in sex anymore. When we try to have sex, it hurts. I feel like an old lady. I have to do something."*

Attention:

Restless sleep and hot flashes are telling you something is missing!

Her primary care physician said it couldn't be her hormones, and told her she was just too stressed and needed to see a therapist.

When I did her evaluation, Susie's levels of estradiol and testosterone were those of someone 80 years old. Even though she was taking estrogen, the horse-derived mixture of estrogens in Premarin does not give much of the human 17-beta estradiol a woman's body makes. This is why she still had so many hot flashes and fragmented sleep. Her low estradiol caused vaginal dryness and difficulty becoming lubricated during sex, making intercourse very painful.

Adding to her problems from low estradiol, her free testosterone level plummeted with the combination of the potent synthetic progestin and the oral estrogen mixture she was taking. No wonder she didn't have any energy… or libido.

I changed her to a bioidentical 17-beta estradiol as her body had always made before menopause. I also suggested she use an estradiol skin patch, which results in higher free testosterone than the oral estrogen she had been using. I expected this change to improve her libido and help her to feel less tired.

To restore her energy level and sex drive back to her usual level, however, she also needed supplemental testosterone to bring the total testosterone level to a desirable range. I added a low dose 0.25 mg/gm cream form of testosterone for her to use every morning, applied to her tummy with a little bit used on the vulva.

The testosterone in the cream is absorbed through the skin into the bloodstream and gives just about the level of testosterone that we would see in a woman in her late twenties.

I also recommended she switch to a bioidentical progesterone using the FDA-approved brand, Prometrium, and suggested that she only use progesterone every two months for 12 days instead of taking a progestin every day as she had been doing. That way, she could pick which twelve days every couple of months that she didn't mind feeling a little slowed down or tired from the progesterone rather than feeling that way every day. She liked the new options and agreed to try them.

At her follow up appointment several months later, she was a very happy camper:

> "I feel just great. The hot flashes are gone and I am sleeping a lot better now. I have a better attitude, I don't feel depressed, I feel like my life is worth living now. I also have better muscle tone with my exercise, I can tell in my legs and arms that my muscle isn't as flabby. My muscles respond better to exercise now. Sex is less painful, there is a big improvement in that area. I can also notice a difference in my libido, and it's easier to have an orgasm. I am feeling really good and I am so glad I came to see you! It has been a big help."

She did not experience any negative side effects or

Heads Up!

What is normal for you is not necessarily normal for someone else.

problems with her new hormone approaches, and said,

> "I can't think of anything that isn't going well. I really like how I feel since you added testosterone, and the estrogen patch is working well. But I can tell when it is wearing off and I need to change it because the hot flashes start coming back and I don't sleep as well. This progesterone is much better and I don't feel so bloated and tired all the time."

She was pleased to hear that her hormone levels had also improved, which convinced her that her symptoms had been due to her low hormone levels as she had suspected all along. When I first saw her, the FSH was clearly menopausal at 146, her estradiol was only 30 pg/ml, total testosterone was only 20 ng/dl, and her free testosterone was undetectable.

At a recent follow up, her FSH had come down to 53 indicating that her brain was registering a better estradiol level in the bloodstream now. Her total testosterone was now up to 47 ng/dl, with a free testosterone of 5.0, about the levels I had hoped to achieve.

Overview of Testosterone's Importance

Testosterone is far more than just "the sex hormone." Testosterone has an impact on every major *system* in our body, from hair to skin to eyes to muscles to bone to brain.

Testosterone affects major *functions*, too: growth, metabolism, immune pathways, mood, sleep, dreaming, appetite...and of course, our sex drive, sexual responsiveness, orgasm.

Women who are now reaching menopausal age naturally are the "tip of the iceberg" of those who need to know more about testosterone and the role it plays in our health.

Below the surface, a larger part of the "iceberg" is made up of surgically menopausal and even perimenopausal

Who is listening?

You know you best. If your doctor isn't listening, find another one! It isn't easy, but it can be done, or... try to educate the one you have.

women, numbering in the millions. These are the women like Kelly, who had a hysterectomy in their 30s and 40s, many years before the typical age of "natural" menopause.

Loss of the ovaries causes more than a 50% loss of testosterone, with a devastating blow to sexual function. Estradiol also drops to barely detectable levels, leading to a further blunting of sexual desire, loss of vaginal lubrication, loss of ability to become aroused during sex, and difficulty reaching orgasm.

Wake UP!

Women have more problems with low libido than men—but men get the help while women are ignored.

Even when the ovaries are left in place, studies show that, on average, women's estradiol and testosterone drop to menopausal levels within 2-3 years after the hysterectomy, regardless of the age at which she has the hysterectomy. Then, because everyone thinks the ovaries are still there and working just fine, no one thinks to check hormone levels to see if they really are "just fine."

So doctors don't find out that low hormone levels can cause such anguish. These women suffer in silence. Or, they are told to take an antidepressant, which makes libido plummet even further.

Even more overlooked is another part of the "iceberg" lying under the surface of women's health. Healthy women in their late 30s and early 40s may have only *half* the levels of testosterone and estradiol they had in their 20's, if they are already among those beginning to have falling hormone levels long before they actually hit the typical age of menopause.

These women have either premature ovarian decline, or actual premature menopause, also called premature ovarian failure.

Even young women taking birth control pills (BCP) can be affected. Many don't realize that the pills have another "contraceptive effect" that no one is talking about—*low sex drive!* That's right.

Birth control pills lower the free, active testosterone

because the oral hormones stimulate the liver to make a protein called *sex hormone binding globulin*, or SHBG. Then SHBG binds up free testosterone and makes it less active. This can be a *benefit* in women with acne or excess body hair due to excess testosterone, such as happens in women with Polycystic Ovarian Syndrome (PCOS).

If a woman has low or normal testosterone levels, however, then higher SHBG causing decreased free testosterone can be a major drawback, resulting in low sex drive, fatigue, blue or blah moods, and achy muscles.

When you put all these groups of women together across many age groups, you can see that there are *millions* of women likely to have diminished sex drive and low energy levels due to low testosterone. The good news is, they can be helped.

Low sexual desire

Research suggests approximately 35-45% of women perceive they have some type of sexual problem, **most commonly low sexual desire**. The 2000 Female Sexual Function Forum meeting reported that almost equal numbers of premenopausal women and postmenopausal women complained of decreased libido.

The 1992 National Health and Social Life Survey surprised researchers with results that showed the prevalence of sexual dysfunction in the United States to be more common in women than men. In fact, the study found that 43% of women between the ages of 18 to 59 had sexual dysfunction compared to 31% of men. *This study estimated the number of women with distressingly low libido to be in the "tens of millions."*

When I attended the International Testosterone Symposium in Germany in the fall of 2003, Dr. Peter Casson, a leading researcher on androgens in women said "I predict that in five to ten years, more women than men will be treated for androgen insufficiency."

Statistics

You are definitely *not* alone!

Fact:

It's real. Speak UP!

Testosterone deficiency is real

Testosterone deficiency is a genuine medical, endocrine condition. It must be taken seriously, and deserves careful medical evaluation.

Far too many women are in despair watching their once healthy energetic bodies slip away and turn to mush. They are distressed that their relationships suffer because they no longer have any interest in sex. They deserve to know that help is available. They need to know that adverse side effects of testosterone are uncommon when the hormone is administered in ways and amounts that mimic our natural ovarian production as closely as possible.

Yet, even today, few doctors discuss testosterone as a treatment option and few women's health books mention testosterone as an important female hormone.

Women have already been talking about it, but using testosterone will be a new idea for most physicians, most of whom don't know how to use it effectively for women.

Because of this, even women who have figured out that they have low testosterone levels frequently struggle with improper dosing and unwanted side effects.

Together women and their physicians will need to learn how to use testosterone optimally for women.

I will teach you more about this in later chapters. For now, let's explore in greater detail about what androgens are, where in our body they are made, and the myriad ways they play critical roles in our sexuality, vitality, and strength.

Chapter 2
Testosterone and Androgens in Women: What They Are and What They Do

What is Testosterone?

Testosterone is one of a group of hormones called *androgens*, from the Greek "andros" meaning "male-like." *Androgen* refers to steroid molecules with 19 carbon atoms (*testosterone, dihydrotestosterone or DHT*) synthesized from cholesterol in the ovaries and adrenal glands that are able to directly bind to and activate the androgen hormone receptor sites throughout the brain and body.

Androgen also refers to 19-carbon molecules *androstene-dione, dehydroepiandrosterone or DHEA, DHEA-sulfate or DHEA-S* made from other building blocks primarily in the ovaries and adrenal glands, and also in the brain, fat tissue, skin, muscle and other tissues.

Androgens can also be made from the estrogen, *estrone,* via the *aromatase* enzyme present in the ovaries, brain, breast, body fat tissue, bone, muscle, and skin. Many of you may not realize that testosterone can also be converted to *estradiol* by the aromatase enzyme in many different tissues.

Testosterone is then converted to DHT by the enzyme, 5α reductase. Skin, for example, often has high amounts of 5α reductase, which explains why high testosterone can cause skin problems like acne and excess hair.

Testosterone and DHT are our primary androgens. Androstenedione, DHEA and DHEA-s are more correctly called *pro-androgens* because they have to *first* be converted to testosterone before they can activate

> **FACT:**
> Most women don't know that *low* testosterone has such a devastating effect on our lives.

Wisdom:

How much testosterone does your body produce?

• About 10 percent of what a healthy man has

• The average amount per day in young women is 200-400 micrograms, half from the ovaries and half from the adrenal glands

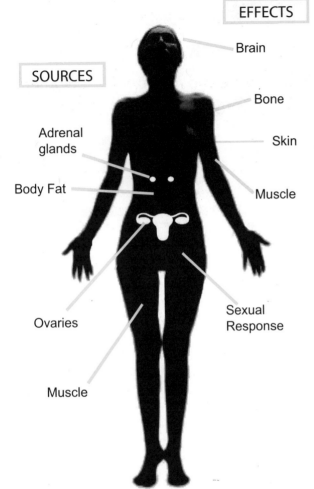

SOURCES

EFFECTS

Adrenal glands

Body Fat

Ovaries

Muscle

Brain

Bone

Skin

Muscle

Sexual Response

TYPES OF ANDROGENS and WHERE PRODUCED

- ঀ Testosterone–ovary, adrenal gland primarily
- ঀ Dihydrotestosterone–ovary, adrenal, body fat, skin
- ঀ Dehydroepiandrosterone (DHEA)–ovary and adrenal
- ঀ Dehydroepiandrosterone sulfate (DHEA-S)–adrenal gland and ovary
- ঀ Androstenedione–ovary, adrenal gland, body fat

androgen receptors to exert full androgenic effects. Since these pro-androgen building blocks are produced in the ovaries and adrenal glands, it really ends up that the ovaries and adrenal glands together are responsible, either directly or indirectly, for making just about all of a woman's testosterone. That's why it can be such a major blow to our sex drive and energy level when the ovaries are removed, damaged, or become menopausal.

The amount of active circulating androgens is obviously much lower in women than in men, only about 1/10th of what a man's body makes. Even though women make so much less testosterone, what we have packs a powerful punch though out our minds and bodies. Testosterone and it's sister androgens are crucial for quite an array of vital functions in women's bodies. Many studies over the last *seventy* years have demonstrated the potent effects of testosterone on a woman's sexual urges, mood, sense of vital energy and psychological well-being. Testosterone also helps build and maintain healthy muscle and bone, and it strengthens the tissues of the vagina and labia, as well as enhancing clitoral nerve sensitivity.

Fact:

The older you get, the more you may need testosterone.

Not surprisingly, in a Gallup poll of American women, conducted for the North American Menopause Society in 1993, only 5% of the women polled knew that their bodies make "androgens," including testosterone that we think of as a "man's" hormone. More than 95% of the women also did not know that androgens declined after menopause. Doctors have also thought that testosterone wasn't very important for women, so the whole idea of testosterone therapy for women is relatively new to physicians today.

Many of you may not know, however, that beginning in the 1940s, a few enlightened pioneers like Dr. Robert Greenblatt in the United States and later Professor Morrie Gelfand in Canada, began using testosterone therapy for women with positive results. About thirty years ago, Canadian Psychologist Dr. Barbara Sherwin systematically studied testosterone effects on sexual function, mood, and cognition again showing how crucial testosterone is for women.

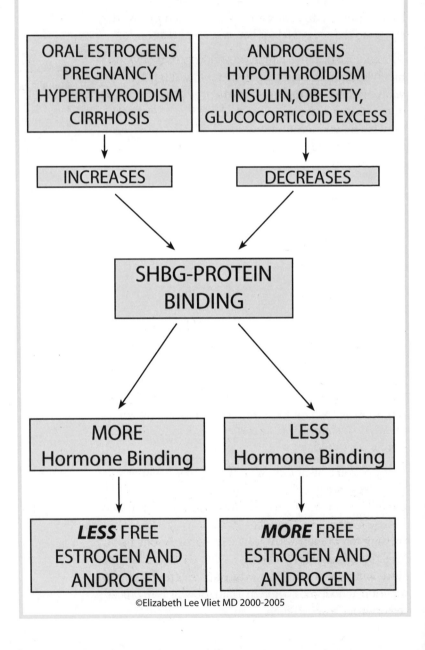

Sex Hormone Binding Globulin (SHBG)
Interactions with Hormones

ORAL ESTROGENS PREGNANCY HYPERTHYROIDISM CIRRHOSIS	ANDROGENS HYPOTHYROIDISM INSULIN, OBESITY, GLUCOCORTICOID EXCESS

INCREASES → → ← DECREASES

SHBG-PROTEIN BINDING

MORE Hormone Binding	LESS Hormone Binding
LESS FREE ESTROGEN AND ANDROGEN	**MORE** FREE ESTROGEN AND ANDROGEN

©Elizabeth Lee Vliet MD 2000-2005

Other physician-researchers today, such as Drs. Phillip Sarrel, Morris Notelovitz and Gloria Bachman in the United States, Professor Andrea Genazzani in Italy, Professors Henry Burger, Susan Davis, and Lorraine Dennerstein in Australia, have been leaders in the field with their studies showing positive effects of adding testosterone to estrogen therapy for both naturally and surgically menopausal women.

As new information emerges from current studies, we have even more understanding of the many ways that our androgens play crucial roles in our overall health. Effects far beyond the obvious sexual ones are being uncovered for women, and for men too.

Fortunately, more women today are aware of the importance of androgens like testosterone and DHEA and are asking physicians for more information about what they do, how to measure these hormones, and what options exist to add back what the body formerly made.

Androgens, especially our testosterone, are *anabolic* hormones. *Anabolic* means "able to build." Anabolic hormones like testosterone use our food and stored body fat for the fuel to build muscle and bone, our lean body mass, also sometimes called "fat-free mass." Women lose more muscle as we age than men do, so it is especially important to have optimal testosterone for women.

Androgens use stored body fat for fuel to build other tissues like muscle and bone, so these important hormones help to decrease our percentage of body fat, a very good thing! Since muscles are our most efficient fat-burning machinery, androgens help us lose excess body fat (a) directly, by using fat stores to build muscle, and (b) indirectly, by creating increased muscle mass that burns more calories twenty-four hours a day, whether we are exercising or not.

All of this happens as long as we have the right balance of androgens and our other metabolic hormones, including estradiol, thyroid, cortisol, and insulin. This is another reason that it is so important to check your testosterone quotient!

Not Too Much!

A tiny bit goes a long way.

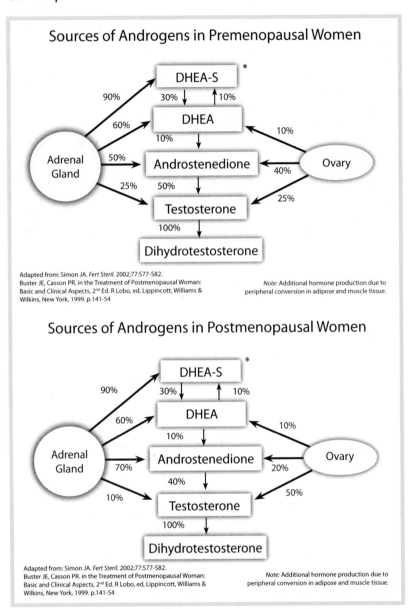

Sources of Androgens in Premenopausal Women

Adapted from: Simon JA. *Fert Steril.* 2002;77:S77-S82.
Buster JE, Casson PR. in the Treatment of Postmenopausal Woman: Basic and Clinical Aspects, 2nd Ed. R Lobo, ed, Lippincott, Williams & Wilkins, New York, 1999. p.141-54

Note: Additional hormone production due to peripheral conversion in adipose and muscle tissue.

Sources of Androgens in Postmenopausal Women

Adapted from: Simon JA. *Fert Steril.* 2002;77:S77-S82.
Buster JE, Casson PR. in the Treatment of Postmenopausal Woman: Basic and Clinical Aspects, 2nd Ed. R Lobo, ed, Lippincott, Williams & Wilkins, New York, 1999. p.141-54

Note: Additional hormone production due to peripheral conversion in adipose and muscle tissue.

Testosterone is a potent hormone. A tiny bit goes a long way. Because it is so potent, most of our testosterone is carried in the bloodstream in an inactive form strongly attached to a carrier protein called *sex hormone binding globulin* (SHBG) that is made in the liver. Only a tiny fraction, about 1-2 % of the total testosterone, circulates in the blood stream in the active, or *free*, form. Free testosterone is the active form, available to instantaneously activate the testosterone receptors throughout the body. Testosterone bound to SHBG is like a storage reservoir, inactive while attached to its carrier, but ready to be released and become active the instant the body needs it.

Testosterone is weakly attached to another carrier protein in the blood called *albumin*. Doctors used to think that only the *free* form was biologically active at testosterone receptors, but in 1991 research found that *both* the free portion *and* the portion weakly bound to albumin are biologically active and able to stimulate the testosterone receptor.

Together, testosterone that is weakly bound *and* free serves as our active, *bioavailable* supply. This means testing ideally should include all three forms in the bloodstream—free, weakly bound, and total testosterone—to give the clearest picture of our available active testosterone.

These new findings also mean that anything that *increases* SHBG *or* albumin will *lower* the active form of testosterone and likely decrease our sex drive, muscle strength, and energy level. Likewise, anything that *lowers* SHBG or albumin will make more of the free testosterone and potentially cause unwanted symptoms of excess testosterone such as facial hair, acne, or disrupted sleep.

Many factors affect the amount of hormone that is "free" at any given time. Some of the most common are shown in the chart that follows.

Other factors include medications that are highly protein bound. Such medications compete for the carrier proteins and move more of the hormone into the free form, possibly producing symptoms of hormone excess. Or the opposite may happen. Some medications will push more of the hormone into the bound and inactive form, leaving less in the free, active fraction. In Chapter 9, I have listed the many different medications that can affect sex drive and sexual responsiveness by a variety of mechanisms, including effects on protein-binding.

Ok, Ok...

Yes, we know it's complicated, but, so are our bodies!

Oral birth control pills (BCP) are a good example of medication that decreases free testosterone. Because they are taken orally, BCP stimulate the liver to make more SHBG, which attaches to testosterone and makes less free testosterone. Women with androgen *excess* find this effect desirable, because it reduces acne, excess facial and body hair. But other women may be very bothered by a drop in libido or energy level after being on "the pill" for several months. I often call this the "overlooked contraceptive effect" of birth control pills —some women lose interest in even having sex! If low libido becomes a problem on oral BCP, you can ask to change to a contraceptive vaginal ring (Nuvaring) or patch (Ortho Evra) since both of these avoid the liver first pass, and don't increase SHBG.

Fact:

It isn't usually the hysterectomy itself that caused the fatigue and loss of sex drive.

It's the loss of estradiol and testosterone.

On the other hand, some conditions like hypothyroidism can *decrease* SHBG and cause *increased* free testosterone and all its usual symptoms. But because hypothyroidism impairs the ovaries' ability to make *all* its hormones that are involved in sexual response, the decline in estradiol, testosterone and DHEA may mean that you don't have an increase in sex drive with the increase in free testosterone sometimes seen in hypothyroidism.

I know it is a complicated picture, but I hope this helps you see how many different factors may affect your level of available testosterone in a variety of ways. It helps you understand why it is so important to your health to carefully evaluate all of this.

The Menstrual Cycle and Testosterone

Testosterone production by the ovary is different from the characteristic cycles of estradiol and progesterone that rise and fall quite dramatically over the course of each menstrual cycle. Testosterone levels tend to be fairly steady throughout the monthly cycle, except that some women experience a brief surge of testosterone around midcycle, when estradiol peaks.

This midcycle rise in testosterone is not seen in all women, even though they have a healthy midcycle rise in estradiol and normal ovulation. Women with fertile menstrual cycles often experience a rise in sexual desire around the time of ovulation, but since both estradiol and testosterone can be rising together at midcycle, the increase in libido may be due to either to both.

Many women report changes in libido at different times of their menstrual cycle. One 1987 study found that women with high normal testosterone levels across the menstrual cycle are less depressed and experience more sexual satisfaction than women with low normal testosterone levels. These changes in our desire for sex probably don't just relate to how much *total* testosterone is present. Libido is also affected by the amount of *free* testosterone circulating in the bloodstream, and by the ability of testosterone to bind to and activate its receptors in the brain and sexual organs. Estradiol fluctuations cause changes in free testosterone. It is the free testosterone that primarily activates the sexual circuits in our brain. When estradiol levels are lower and there is a larger amount of free testosterone, we may experience increased sex drive, unless estradiol is too low.

> **Warning**
>
> Proper treatment can't begin without proper blood tests. Insist on them!

Intensity of sex drive can also be affected by the rise in estradiol and by rise and fall in progesterone. Progesterone is an "*inhibitor*" of testosterone, and decreases testosterone binding at its receptors, which in turn will decrease desire for sex. This may be one reason so many women describe having low libido during the "PMS" week, when progesterone peaks and blocks testosterone activity.

My own work tracking hormone levels in women of many ages, correlated with their reported symptoms, suggests that hormonal action to enhance sexual desire involves (1) adequate levels of both estradiol and testosterone, particularly in the free forms, and (2) testosterone present in optimal balance with estradiol to have their complimentary effects on sexual response. I find that the *ratio* of these hormones, and the balance with DHEA, is critically important to maintain healthy sex drive and sexual responsiveness for women. Along this

Dr. Vliet's Guide to the Menstrual Cycle Hormone Rhythm

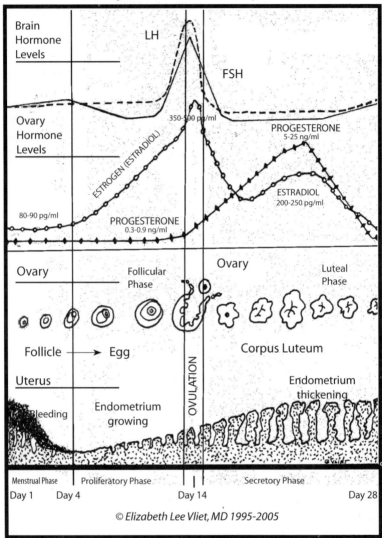

© Elizabeth Lee Vliet, MD 1995-2005

same line, more recent studies using a testosterone patch for surgically and naturally menopausal women taking estrogen found that restoring testosterone to high normal ranges gave significant improvement in sexual desire. This beneficial effect on sex drive wasn't seen in most women taking oral estrogen alone. Even better results occurred when women used a patch form of estradiol instead of oral estrogen.

Follicular Phase: When Estradiol is Dominant

Estradiol is the dominant hormone of the first half of the menstrual cycle, from menses onset to ovulation, or approximately day 1 to about day 14. There are two peaks of estradiol in our monthly cycles: a rise to the peak just before ovulation, then an abrupt drop, and another smaller rise after ovulation when progesterone peaks. Mood-elevating and energizing effects of estradiol are much more pronounced the first half of the menstrual cycle, as estradiol is rising before ovulation, while progesterone is still quite low. If the rise in estradiol during the second half (luteal phase) of the menstrual cycle isn't enough to give the optimal balance with progesterone, I find in my patients that this is what triggers more PMS, irritability, lethargy, bloating, depressed mood, and loss of sex drive. That really isn't surprising, since progesterone acts as a central nervous system depressant, and binds at the same brain receptor as Valium, a known culprit in low libido, depressed mood and tiredness. If there isn't enough estradiol, or testosterone, to give mood-lifting effects as a balance to the "downer" effects of progesterone, then it's no wonder you get irritable and depressed!

Wisdom:

Testosterone typically peaks at mid-cycle.

Luteal Phase: When Progesterone is Dominant

At ovulation, the dominant follicle pops off into the space between the ovary and Fallopian tube, and becomes the "egg" or *corpus luteum*, which begins pumping out progesterone to prepare the uterus to receive and nourish a fertilized egg until the placenta takes over hormone production. This rise in progesterone peaks about the 20th day following the beginning of your last bleeding. Progesterone thickens the uterine lining and stimulates accelerated growth of breast tissue. In addition, progesterone prepares a woman's body to adapt to the many metabolic and physical demands of pregnancy. It increases appetite, triggers more water retention, sets off cravings for certain foods (chocolate, anyone?), and increases oil secretion in the skin, making acne flares more likely. Progesterone's sedative effects make us slowed down and sleepy, while it's testosterone-blocking effects make us less interested in sex. Progesterone's immune suppressing effects make yeast infections or herpes outbreaks more likely.

Premenstrual Phase: Falling hormones

If fertilization does not occur, there is no pregnancy, so the corpus luteum withers away, stops making progesterone and progesterone levels fall over the next several days. The thickened uterine lining that wasn't needed for a new embryo is shed in menstrual bleeding to make ready for the next cycle. The corpus luteum is also the primary source of estradiol during the luteal phase, so as it withers and dies, there is a drop in estradiol before menses too.

It is the *drop in progesterone* that triggers the shedding of the uterine lining to start menses. The *drop in estradiol* can trigger such problems as hot flashes, restless fragmented sleep, migraine headaches, vaginal dryness. The fall in both hormones affect chemical messengers in the brain that regulate mood, so that's why you may notice mood changes around the first few days of bleeding. I have shown the estradiol and progesterone changes in the preceding menstrual cycle chart.

Pay attention to the physical, emotional, and sexual changes that you experience month to month, then track those changes with the chart of typical hormone changes I have shown. This will give you an idea of hormone connections in the body changes you experience each cycle.

The Testosterone Life Cycle

Over the course of a woman's life, the ovary makes on average about one-third or more of a woman's total androgens, and about half of her testosterone, in addition to producing estrogen, estrone, progesterone, and DHEA. During our reproductive life, the ovaries and adrenal glands produce about 0.3 milligrams of testosterone per day, on average. Beginning several years before a woman's ovary becomes menopausal, the adrenal glands have already decreased androgen production by about 50%, and the ovary levels of testosterone have also started to decrease.

One study found that mean testosterone levels for women at age 21 was about *two times higher* than levels in women at age 40. In the Study of Women's Health Across the Nation (SWAN), researchers found approximately a 25% decrease in testosterone between age 42 and 50. Since the average age for ending of menses, or menopause, is 51, that means your sexual desire and ability to become sexually aroused, as well as your energy level, can be significantly diminished several years *before you actually stop having periods.*

Heads UP!

Losing your stamina? Check your hormones!

Most women know that menopause brings the loss of "estrogen," but most do not realize that even with natural menopause, there is also a loss of *androgens,* including diminished testosterone. One reason testosterone declines after menopause is that an important precursor molecule *androstenedione,* decreases more than 50 percent when the ovary fades out of hormone production. The other major androgen precursors, DHEA and DHEA-S, drop sharply after age 35. Loss of these precursors means our bodies can't make as much testosterone during the years leading up to menopause and afterwards.

"Perimenopausal" decrease in hormones can occur in some women in their mid thirties, for other women it happens in their forties, and for still others, the decline doesn't hit until their fifties. This means it may be hard to know when the decline in testosterone actually begins for women unless hormone levels are actually measured.

I think this is why so many doctors today do not realize how many clinical symptoms women describe are due to the loss of estradiol and testosterone, or just how much testosterone women lose around the time we have a decline in our ovarian hormone levels.

Natural Menopause

There is a critical difference between the way testosterone production occurs in women vs. men: ovaries lose their major "hormone-producing factories" when a woman's supply of follicles ("eggs") is used up, but men's testicles are able to keep making sperm and hormones their entire lives. This is the primary reason that menopause in women comes sooner and has more dramatic changes: there is a sharper fall in women's hormones than the gradual decline seen in men that also tends to occur at a much later age. One exception is men who drink alcohol daily. Alcohol decreases testosterone production in the testicle and also increases the metabolism of testosterone to estrone, which causes men to develop unwanted estrogen effects such as breasts (*gynecomastia*).

Warning:

Testosterone in balance with estradiol is crucial.

Men may not lose 50% of their testosterone until their late 70s or early 80s. Women, on the other hand, lose about 50% of their testosterone in their 40s and 50s, *ten to twenty years ahead of when men begin to experience similar problems.* I have often wondered if women's loss of hormones so much sooner than men is one reason many men leave long-standing marriages and turn to younger women around this time. Men often don't know what is happening to their wives causing less sexual interest. They begin to take it personally, and seek satisfaction elsewhere. Tragically, doctors often make this problem worse by prescribing antidepressants for the woman, making her even *less* sexually responsive, while the man gets Viagra to make *his* sexual performance better! No wonder marriages often fly apart in midlife.

Surgical Menopause

If you have a hysterectomy *with* removal of the ovaries before you are actually menopausal, the change is even more drastic. Concentrations of testosterone in the bloodstream fall markedly *within twenty-four to forty-eight hours* after surgery. Since you no longer have the ovaries to make more testosterone, or to convert adrenal hormones (DHEA) to testosterone, there is an abrupt loss of this important hormone. That's a big shock to the body.

There are potentially major unpleasant effects from the loss of testosterone: loss of sex drive, fatigue, decrease in muscle mass, decreased bone density, depressed mood, achy joints, and changes in feelings of well-being, to name a few. Even if one or both ovaries are left in place, newer studies have shown that the hormone production reaches menopausal levels within 3-4 years for as many as 60 to 70 percent of women, even if they are only in their thirties when the uterus is removed.

Wisdom:

Even if not removed, ovaries decrease hormone production sooner after hysterectomy

This more rapid decline in hormones after the uterus is removed is thought to be due to decreased blood flow to the ovaries as a result of having to cut and tie off the uterine artery during surgery. The ovaries don't function as well with reduced blood flow and less oxygen available to make your hormones. That means hormone ratios change, PMS tends to get worse, and you begin to have more and more menopausal symptoms, along with a disappearing libido.

If you are then started on oral estrogen therapy like the commonly used Premarin, the amount of free, biologically active testosterone falls even further. This is because oral estrogen increases liver manufacture of SHBG that "binds up" more of the testosterone molecules, leaving less testosterone available for the body to use. This is one reason that many women lose interest in sex, or don't lubricate as well, or find that orgasm is harder to reach, as well as have more fatigue after hysterectomy.

They often blame the surgery, but it isn't usually the surgery itself that caused these problems; it's the loss of optimal estradiol and testosterone leading to fatigue and loss of sex drive. To keep more of the remaining testosterone in the free, active form, it really helps to use estradiol in a non-oral form, like Estrasorb lotion or a patch, instead of Premarin pills.

To feel as well as you did before hysterectomy and removal of the ovaries, you need to restore both hormones to optimal ranges for your body as you had before surgery. *Most* women who have had their ovaries removed will need testosterone *plus* estradiol, but only about 5% of women actually get a testosterone included in their prescriptions. Even with as much as we know today about the many roles testosterone plays in women's mind-body health, most doctors don't think to add back the lost testosterone component of a woman's hormone makeup.

Warning:

Both prescription and over the counter medications can decrease your hormone levels and blunt sex drive.

Many times after hysterectomy, doctors attribute low energy, loss of sex drive and blah mood to "depression" and recommend antidepressants. And when you start an SSRI, your libido can *really* plummet, along with your ability to have an orgasm. Except for Wellbutrin (buproprion), *all* of the antidepressants in use today (serotonin-augmenting ones, tricyclics, MAO inhibitors, and most of the "mood stabilizers") have potentially disastrous results for your sex life.

Serotonin-augmenting medications, or SSRIs (Zoloft, Paxil, Celexa, Lexapro, Prozac, Luvox), are particularly notorious for drastically reducing sex drive and making it hard or impossible to have an orgasm. This happens in women who have *normal* levels of testosterone. The effect is much worse for women who have *low* testosterone.

How do doctors really know *what* you need if no one ever checks hormone levels before or after surgery, or even considers that loss of crucial hormones may cause loss of libido, depressed mood, and fatigue?

Women and Androgen Insufficiency Syndrome (AIS)

The concept of a clinical syndrome of *androgen insufficiency* in women is not a new idea. As early as 1938, Drs. Shorr, Papanicolaou and Stimmel observed that adding "male sex hormone" to menopausal women helped improve women's sexual interest. In 1940, Dr.

Loeser described increased sexual drive after women received subcutaneous implants of both male and female hormones.

Dr. Robert Greenblatt, a pioneer in the use and effects of estrogens and androgens in men and women, described testosterone as "the only true aphrodisiac." He published numerous studies showing the many benefits of androgens for women. Many other physicians around this time were also finding that testosterone helped improve sexual function and mood in menopausal women, or women who had undergone removal of the ovaries. Studies also described effects of androgens on muscle strength and energy level. Later, Dr. Barbara Sherwin conducted a series of ground breaking research studies showing combined estrogen-androgen therapy had cognitive as well as sexual benefits.

Fact:

Symptoms of low testosterone overlap those of low E2 or low thyroid

Over the years, this cluster of clinical symptoms from loss of androgens has been called *Female Androgen Deficiency* (FAD) or *Female Androgen Insufficiency* (FAI).

In 2001, The Princeton Conference, composed of distinguished physicians and androgen researchers from several countries, was convened in Princeton, New Jersey to review the worldwide data on the role of androgens in women to look at what we know, and what still needs to be clarified. As an outgrowth of The Princeton Conference, *Androgen Insufficiency Syndrome* became the term we now use to describe the symptoms and bodily changes that occur with androgen loss in women.

The following tables represent key findings from published studies on androgen insufficiency in women, in addition to descriptions from my clinical experience over the years doing evaluations of women with low testosterone.

I think it is striking how many symptoms overlap those described for *clinical major depression*. We seem the same symptom overlap between low estradiol, hypothyroidism and major depression. It seems to me only common sense that we can't very well know *which* problem to treat if no one measures a woman's hormone levels! Even if they do help lift mood, antidepressants certainly don't correct all the physical problems caused by low thyroid, low estradiol *or* low testosterone…and may even make the problems worse! So if you are experiencing some of the symptoms and body changes below, make sure you see about getting your hormone levels properly checked.

ANDROGEN INSUFFICIENCY SYNDROME (AIS)

Symptoms—described by women:

- Low or absent libido (sexual desire)
- Low or absent desire to be intimate
- Loss of sexual thoughts, fantasies, dreams
- Diminished sensitivity to sexual stimulation (e.g. clitoris)
- Loss of motivation, diminished assertiveness
- Fatigue/tiredness
- Lethargy/loss of vital energy not explained by other disorders
- Diminished memory, concentration and focus
- Flat, blah mood
- Diminished sense of well-being

Signs—seen on physical exam:

- Diminished body hair (arms, legs, underarms)
- Thinning and loss of pubic hair
- Diminished clitoral size
- Thinning of labia
- Diminished muscle mass and strength
- Bone loss (seen on DEXA)

© Elizabeth Lee Vliet, M.D. 2001-2005

What Causes Low Androgens, especially Testosterone, in Women?

There are many different ways that our androgen production can be adversely affected, from problems affecting the ovaries, to adrenal and thyroid or pituitary disorders, to medications, and to lifestyle choices. Let's look at few and a brief explanation of why they cause low testosterone.

Getting older is the most common reason women lose testosterone. As we age, we lose ovarian follicles that are our main hormone producing factories. Menopause is the time frame that leads to profound loss of androgen precursors made by the ovaries, in addition to the loss of estradiol.

But young women also lose of testosterone for a variety of reasons. Vegan diets are often low in protein and a number of important vitamins and minerals, and have been shown consistently to reduce ovarian hormone levels in young women. Dieting to lose weight and becoming too thin can cause decline in ovarian hormones.

Hysterectomy with removal of the ovaries is a common cause for younger women to lose testosterone. Removing the ovaries during surgery dramatically drops testosterone by 50 to 80 percent of a presurgical level. Even when the ovaries are left after removing the uterus, disruption of ovarian blood flow can cause significant loss of testosterone and estradiol within 2-3 years of surgery.

Damage to the ovaries from viral and other illnesses, endometriosis, cancer chemotherapy, radiation therapy, environmental endocrine disruptors (e.g., pesticides, dioxin, etc.), toxins, pelvic surgery, and possibly even tubal ligation can also lead to low testosterone in younger women.

Autoimmune illnesses cause diminished ovarian hormone production. Autoimmune illnesses can also disrupt adrenal androgen production, compounding the loss of ovarian androgens. Autoimmune thyroid-

Wisdom:

Even tubal ligation can lower hormone levels

itis, such as Hashimoto's thyroiditis (hypothyroidism) or Graves' disease (hyperthyroidism) damage thyroid hormone production, which in turn leads to ovarian dysfunction and ovarian hormone loss. Hypopituitarism and adrenal failure (Addison's disease) can also cause low testosterone production.

A variety of medications can cause low testosterone production due to effects on brain neurotransmitters needed for sexual desire and arousal. Serotonin boosters (like Prozac, Paxil, Luvox, Zoloft, Celexa, Lexapro) increase serotonin and dampen sexual response. All of the SSRIs listed above, as well as other classes of antidepressant, antipsychotic and mood stabilizer medications can cause elevated prolactin that will suppress normal ovarian hormone levels. Birth control pills also decrease ovarian production of testosterone and DHEA, as well as decreasing the amount of free testosterone by stimulating the liver to make more SHBG.

Fact:

Cholesterol can be pushed too low... and decrease your testosterone!

Statin medicines (Lipitor, Crestor, Pravachol, Zocor, etc.) can lower testosterone production in both women and men because they decrease cholesterol, which is the primary building block needed to make testosterone. In the focus on lowering cholesterol to help prevent heart disease, many doctors don't realize that lowering cholesterol *also* lowers libido!

Oral menopausal hormone preparations increase SHBG and lower testosterone. This problem more pronounced with mixed equine or esterified estrogens like Premarin, Cenestin, or Estratab. Even the oral bioidentical 17-beta estradiol tablets can increase SHBG, but to a lesser extent, because the amount given is usually less than the total estrogen load in the mixed estrogen products. Oral combined estrogen-progestin products, such as Prempro, pack a double whammy because they contain the progestin medroxyprogesterone acetate (MPA) that blocks testosterone action at receptors, *in addition* to the loss of free testosterone caused by oral estrogen effects on SHBG. Women taking any of these products should have both total and free testosterone levels checked in order to determine an optimal amount of testosterone to take.

Adrenal corticosteroids decrease ovarian production of testosterone and estradiol. These medications are widely used to treat asthma, allergies and arthritis. In addition to disrupting ovarian function, these medications also decrease adrenal androgen production, resulting in low levels of DHEA that aggravate the loss of testosterone.

Pituitary tumors produce excess prolactin and lower testosterone. Although such tumors are usually benign, they cause problems from over-production of prolactin that acts to inhibit ovarian cycling and ovarian hormone production. Medication such as bromocriptine can block excess prolactin and help restore healthy sexual function.

Nursing decreases androgens and estradiol. High prolactin helps maintain milk flow for nursing mothers, but it suppresses ovarian cycling and hormone production. So, it isn't just a new baby that makes your sex drive disappear! It's also the prolactin triggering reduced testosterone and estradiol levels. Prolactin primarily suppresses a woman's *desire* for sex, rather than her ability to respond once sex is started. Sometimes, however, prolactin is high enough with nursing that it causes so much suppression of estradiol and testosterone that you have vaginal dryness and reduced clitoral sensitivity that make sex painful.

Daily alcohol intake in women interferes with ovarian hormone production to decrease estradiol and testosterone, as well as causing irregular cycles, and increasing the risk of infertility. Alcohol also decreases production of testosterone in men. Heavy alcohol use also leads to higher estrone that in turn increases SHBG, which blunts sex drive by lowering free testosterone. Alcohol depresses the central nervous system, and prevents men from having erections and makes it harder for women and men to have an orgasm.

Wisdom

Nursing is good for the baby... but can lower your hormones and sex drive.

Be patient.

Cigarette smoking causes damage to the ovarian follicles, resulting in loss of testosterone, estradiol, progesterone and DHEA. Women who smoke typically become menopausal several years earlier than non-smokers.

Case Study

Mrs. H—Revitalization after 60

Mrs. H., came to see me for a consult to see if her hormones needed adjusting. She was a delightful, chipper woman in her early sixties who loved to ski every winter, but she had noticed a significant decrease in her stamina and energy on the slopes over the past two or three seasons. She mentioned that she had experienced a noticeable decline in her strength and endurance for skiing. She had never had anyone check her hormone levels, although she had asked several times about having this done.

When I measured her hormones, her estradiol was too low even with her Premarin 0.625 mg. Her testosterone level was so low it could barely be detected, at less than 10 ng/dl. No wonder her energy and strength had declined. I suggested she add testosterone to her therapy, and I also changed her to a bioidentical form of 17-beta estradiol, using a skin patch delivery. She began using 2.5 mg of natural micronized testosterone oral sustained release capsules, along with the Climara transdermal estradiol patch, 0.1mg every 5 days, and has now been on this combination for the past several years. She did not need to take progesterone since she had a hysterectomy many years ago.

Within the first six months, she described a marked increase in her energy level, and said *"I feel like my old spark is coming back."*

The next year at her follow-up visit she gleefully told me that when she returned to the ski slopes that winter after starting testosterone, her ski instructor commented on the noticeable improvements in her strength and stamina. He asked her what her new training regimen had been over the summer. She smiled and said, *"I never told him what really made the difference, but I know it was the testosterone. I could feel my muscles getting stronger with the exercise, and this was different from the way my muscle strength developed when I was just on the Premarin!"* She didn't have any adverse side effects on this dose of testosterone, and her cholesterol profile has continued to be in a healthy range. She also commented,

> *"I just felt better. It's hard to describe, but I just have such a good change in my overall feeling of well-being and energy again. I didn't realize I had lost some of that until I got it back! I really feel like my usual self."*

Wisdom

It's never too late to have a better sex drive and more energy!

Dr. Vliet's Guide to Causes of Low Androgens

- ઝ Getting older
- ઝ Removal of ovaries
- ઝ Damage to ovaries
- ઝ Many medications
- ઝ Prolonged, severe stress
- ઝ Pituitary disorders
- ઝ Autoimmune illnesses
- ઝ Prolonged nursing
- ઝ Extreme thinness
- ઝ Vegetarian (especially vegan) diets
- ઝ Anorexia/Bulimia
- ઝ Obesity
- ઝ Daily alcohol use
- ઝ Cigarette smoking
- ઝ A combination of these factors

© Elizabeth Lee Vliet, M.D. 2001-2005

Summary

Androgens are crucial and powerful hormones affecting our entire being, from head to toe. They aren't just "male" hormones. Present in larger amounts than estrogen during our entire reproductive lives, testosterone plays a dominant role in many functions in women's bodies. Our entire psychological sense of well-being is enhanced by testosterone. In some women, what at first appeared to be depression turned out to be a deficiency of testosterone.

Androgen loss leaves us feeling dragged out, blah, blue, and excessively tired, and lacking the spark of motivation we once had. Yes, this hormone does lift moods and relive depression when the amounts are present at normal levels for women.

But at the other end of the spectrum, if testosterone levels get to be too high for a woman, whether from over-production in the body or from taking excessive amounts of supplemental testosterone, it can make you anxious, agitated, and irritable and cause violent dreams and/or nightmares, difficulty falling asleep, plus the many other unwanted physical changes I have already mentioned.

For women especially, testosterone in *balance* with estradiol is crucial.

As you see, there are many different ways that your testosterone and other androgens can be diminished and affect your energy, sexual function, and vitality. You may not have even realized the many ways this can happen, or what you can do about it.

Let's turn to chapter 3 and 4 and look at some of the other ways that both excess testosterone as well as loss of testosterone can affect you—from the obvious to the not so obvious. Then in later chapters, I will describe at ways to help you regain a healthy balance.

Wisdom

Androgens are powerful hormones.

Make sure yours are in balance.

Summary: Key Testosterone Effects

What does testosterone do?

- ᕽ Stimulates increase in sexual desire

- ᕽ Restores sexual dreams, thoughts, fantasies

- ᕽ Improves clitoral sensitivity

- ᕽ Improves muscle strength

- ᕽ Helps maintain better muscle/fat balance

- ᕽ Helps build bone and prevent bone loss

- ᕽ Maintains normal energy level

- ᕽ Improves sense of well-being

- ᕽ Regulates hair growth on body and scalp

- ᕽ Helps improve immune function

- ᕽ Helps prevent hot flashes and headaches

Chapter 3

Testosterone and Women's Sexuality

"Testosterone is the only true aphrodisiac."
—R. B. Greenblatt, M.D., 1983

"Menopause has been hell, I've gone downhill since last August. I can't think about a new relationship. My body feels dead. I have no sex drive. I don't know if I will ever get back to normal."

Barb, age 44, divorced

"I am having all these night sweats and funny tingling feelings. I don't feel like myself. I feel flat emotionally and very blah. I've lost all my interest in sex and I used to enjoy it so. I mentioned all this to my Gyn and he just gave me an antidepressant. That made my libido totally disappear, and now I can't even have an orgasm at all."

Kate, age 49, married

"I just don't have any desire for sex. I feel terrible about this. I would like to be interested in it, I love my husband and I am very attracted to him. I enjoy sex when we have it, but I just don't feel interested. It frustrates me and it frustrates my husband. It's like somebody turned off a switch."

Mary, age 33, married

"I have a new husband, I love him, and we want to enjoy our sex. I just don't seem to have the inter-est I used to, and it hurts because I'm so dry. My

gynecologist just seemed to dismiss my concerns. He said that's what happens when you get older. I don't want to lose the sexual part of my life."

Thelma, age 67, newly married

"*I became sexually active this past year and went on Alesse for birth control about six months ago. Now I have no sex drive at all, I don't even feel interested in having sex anymore. I don't get lubricated like I used to, and now even if I have sex, it really hurts. I'm too young for this.*"

Laurie, age 24, single

Wisdom:

Before you accept a diagnosis of "it's all in your head," have your hormone levels checked.

All of them!

It's NOT All in Your Head

What happened to each of these women that robbed them of their sexual interest and ability to become aroused and enjoy sex? Each of them came to see me for an evaluation of these problems. They all had questions about hormones, and whether hormone changes could be playing a role in the recent onset of the sexual difficulties.

These women had not been able to get their physicians to do any hormone testing to help them identify a possible underlying cause of their loss of desire. All of these women had been told that they were depressed, needed to take an antidepressant, and to see a therapist to work on their relationship issues.

What about "hormones and sex?" What about testosterone in particular, and estradiol? Don't they *also* play a role in women's sexual desire and arousal?

The answer is a resounding YES. Loss of these critical "sexual activators" causes many different types of sexual problems.

You have all seen the ads for medications that help men's erectile dysfunction. Men are not typically being offered antidepressants as a treatment for ED. That is a big change from my medical school days when ED was considered to be caused by *psychological conflicts*

95% of the time. We now know that ED is caused by hormone problems and various medical disorders in about 90-95% of cases.

Slowly but surely, there is more recognition that women's sexual dysfunction is also a "real" medical issue, not just a psychological problem "in your head." Sexual problems of various types affect *millions* of women. In a study in this country 2900 men and women between the ages of 18 and 60 years were asked about the prevalence of sexual dysfunction. Approximately 24% of the women reported inability to achieve orgasm, 19% reported problems with a lack of lubrication, and 14% reported pain during sex. Another study found that over 40% of women had low sexual desire.

All these sexual problems in women have major hormonal and physical causes that should be properly assessed and diagnosed before the *right* treatment can be identified. If a doctor assumes that it is simply "depression" as the cause and prescribes an antidepressant, it can actually make these problems *worse*.

Let's explore women's sexual response and the many intertwining factors that influence our *interest* in having sex, as well as our ability to become aroused and *enjoy* it. But before I explain the biology of our ability to respond sexually, let's look at some underlying cultural myths and misunderstandings about women's sexuality. Many are alive and well today.

Myths and Stereotypes of Women's Sexuality

For generations, the standard medical teaching was that it was *abnormal* for women to have a sex drive. Women ("good girls" and "ladies") were supposed to be passive recipients of the sex act and were considered "loose" if they appeared to actually *desire* sex.

Even in our sexually explicit culture today, many of these myths and age-old stereotypes lie just beneath the surface in women's encounters with health profes-

Fact:

Our requirements for testosterone may be less than men, but it is still essential to our sexuality!

sionals. I know that seems like a strange idea, given how openly sex is talked about everywhere today. But these hidden messages about women's sexuality, and how women are "supposed" to act are deeply embedded in our culture and especially in the traditional medical teachings.

Take a look at these examples. Some are from a very long time ago and some are more recent, but notice how similar the ideas remain.

Amazing:

Hard to believe this was medical wisdom as *recently* as the 1970s.

Consider these quotes from the textbook of gynecology that we used in 1977 when I was in medical school. That seems like quite a while ago now, but stop and think about all the physicians my age, and even younger, who are practicing medicine today and were trained at the time such textbooks were in use. Here is what the author wrote about libido in women: (bold is my addition)

> "There seems to be little doubt that libido, which is well-developed among normal males, appears to be less highly developed among females. Certainly the majority of cases of dyspareunia [painful intercourse] or frigidity, or both, undoubtedly fall into the **psychogenic** category. The treatment for frigidity must usually stress the educational and psychotherapeutic aspects **rather than the patient's pelvic or endocrine [hormonal] status**.

> "The female should be advised to allow her male partner's sex drive to set their pace and she should attempt to gear hers satisfactorily to his....The importance of the [sex] act to her husband in both physical and emotional aspects should be stressed [i.e. by the physician]."

Viewed from our perspective today, this emphasis on a man's sexual needs being met, and a woman's sexual problems as primarily psychogenic, seems strikingly sexist and unbalanced.

Sadly, these attitudes persist and influence physicians today when women seek help for sexual problems, whether they see a male or a female physician. Just look at the quotes at the beginning of this chapter. These were *not* patients from my medical school days! These were all women I have seen *recently* for consults. There has been a consistent focus on the *psychological* aspects of sexuality for women, while at the same time, for men's sexual desire and arousal, a *physical* model dominates our thinking.

As another example from December 2004, a national TV talk show personality interviewed a *female* psychologist who specializes in treating women with sexual problems. The psychologist, on national television, expressed agreement with the FDA's December 2, 2004 decision to delay approval of *Intrinsa,* the new testosterone patch for women. The psychologist went on to complain that the company seeking FDA approval was *medicalizing* sexual dysfunction, and would increase profits by marketing it to other groups of women once the FDA approved it for women who had undergone hysterectomy and removal of their ovaries.

Excuse me?

Is this psychologist saying that women who have been effectively *castrated* and have no ovaries also have no right to a safe, effective product to restore their lost testosterone?

Is this psychologist saying that it's wrong to offer such a product to other women who might have sexual problems from a loss of testosterone for other reasons?

Do we keep a hormone product off the market for *all* because it *might* be used for someone who may not really need it? Is it wrong to "medicalize" something that clearly can be caused by medical disorders or endocrine imbalance?

I think not.

This statement was made by a psychologist who does not have a medical degree, cannot order blood tests of hormones, cannot do a physical exam to look for physical

> **Wisdom:**
>
> Sexual dysfunction needs to be viewed as a physical, hormonal *and* emotional.

causes of sexual problems, and cannot prescribe medications. Yet, she condemns the use of a testosterone patch to help those women for whom this may be perfectly appropriate to correct the underlying cause of sexual problems.

It's up to a *medical doctor* to properly assess *medical* factors that can cause sexual problems for patients, identify the people for whom testosterone or other hormone therapy is appropriate, and then monitor the patient to be sure she is getting the benefits and not having adverse side effects.

It's time for change:

As you can see, the double standard is alive and well in 2005.

I was appalled that such a negative message about testosterone, a hormone critical to women's bodies, was carried to millions of women around the country, women like those I see every day in my practice who have often suffered for years because no one took them seriously about hormone factors contributing to their difficulties. I wrote the producer to air the "other side" of the story, and to interview women who had been dramatically helped with adding testosterone to their therapy. No response. Stereotypes persist: psychology has the answers for women, hormones to stimulate sexual desire are off limits.

Too many women are being overly *psychologized* and not getting the help that medical treatment options could offer. Women could benefit in major ways by having their testosterone restored to healthy ranges. In my opinion, we very much need to have reliable testosterone product options, such as a patch or pill, available to help women feel their best and regain their sexual spark.

Once again, a psychologist (and now a woman, at that) appears to be saying that women with low testosterone and loss of their sexual desire have no right to seek options other than psychotherapy to help the problem.

Would we do that to men? Of course not. Men already have bioidentical testosterone available in FDA-approved testosterone gel *and* patches in doses right for *male* bodies.

Do women deserve any less?

It sounds to me like we are not that far away from what Dr. W.W. Bliss wrote in 1870, when he warned against a woman having intercourse with "any spasmodic convulsion" (i.e. orgasm) to avoid interfering with conception. He made a rigid distinction between a woman's *reproductive* ability and a woman's *sexuality*. Female sexuality was seen as unwomanly and detrimental to their primary role and function of reproduction.

Dr. Mary Wood-Allen, a woman physician of the same era, taught that women were not meant to enjoy the sex act, and a "ladylike" woman should certainly never *initiate* the sexual act. Dr. Allen wrote that women should embrace their husbands "without a particle of desire."

Physicians during the late 1800s and early 1900s downplayed the existence of women's sexual feelings and desires, but also wrote as if there were an undercurrent of male fear of women's potentially *insatiable lust*, which, if ever aroused, might then become uncontrollable. Could that irrational fear be just under the surface even today?

Look again at the comments from my recent patients shown at the beginning of this chapter. Today, we are dealing with physicians who don't feel it is important to check hormone levels for *women* having problems reaching orgasm.

Yet, it is standard practice to check testosterone *in men* with erectile dysfunction. Doctors either refer women with sexual complaints to therapists for counseling, or assume women are depressed and need antidepressants. *Rarely* do men with sexual problems get prescribed *antidepressants*. Men get prescriptions for testosterone or Viagra or Levitra or Cialis.

Women are *still* getting short shrift when they suffer from sexual problems.

Day in and day out, I hear such stories from women seeking hormone evaluations. I have formal training in

---

Yo! What's wrong with this picture?

Men get Rx for testosterone and Viagra;

Women get Rx for Anti-depressants!

being able to assess the psychological and relationship issues. I spent a year on the sexual consultation team at Johns Hopkins during my residency in the early 1980s, and had extensive training in comprehensive assessment of sexual disorders in men and women. Even at this world-class program, seeing patients from all over the world, we checked *men's* hormone levels as part of the evaluation. We rarely ever checked *women's* hormones, except for thyroid and cortisol.

Fact:

Hormones do help many women immensely, as my patients tell me: "It's like someone turned the light switch back on! I just feel better."

Clearly, the psychological and relationship issues are critical to understand if we are to help our patients. But an *integrated* approach means we can't overlook the *medical*. The focus for *women* is all too often *only* on the psychological, overlooking completely the equally critical functions played by our hormones and other physical factors.

When my patients have asked other medical doctors about hormone testing, they all too often get told "That's not necessary. It won't tell us anything."

I disagree.

When I checked the hormone levels for each of the women quoted at the beginning of this chapter, every one of them had markedly low estradiol levels (most were *less than 30* pg/ml, while a desirable level would be at least 80 to 90 pg/ml), and their testosterone levels were all less than 20 ng/dl (optimal for women is about 40 to 60 ng/dl). These are profound losses of critical hormones.

It helped validate for each woman that because her hormone levels were low, the sexual difficulties they were experiencing were not due to a relationship prob-lem or their "fault." It also helped my patients talk with their husbands. Once the hormone connection was explained, the men didn't feel their wives' loss of desire meant they were lousy lovers. You can appreciate how much relief these couples felt. They also felt hopeful that the problem could be treated.

It is not reasonable to ignore these hormone aspects,

and dismiss a patient's request for a perfectly appropriate blood test, particularly when problems that are identified may be greatly alleviated with available hormone options.

Before physicians send women to therapists, I think it is important to let patients know that (1) we do have reliable and useful tests to measure hormone levels, and (2) we have a variety of bioidentical hormone options to enhance sexual responsiveness once a hormone problem is identified.

Novel thought:

We should check hormones levels, just as we do glucose, cholesterol and thyroid.

After being started on a low dose of supplemental testosterone and estradiol, the 67-year old Thelma came back two months later and said, "*I feel like a new woman. I have my old spark back, and now I want—and enjoy—sex again.*"

Thelma said she no longer had difficulty with arousal and lubrication, her orgasms were now easier to reach and more intense. At the follow up visit, her estradiol level was 98 pg/ml, and her testosterone level was now 45 ng/dl, both good levels for her. The positive change in lab results fit with her self-reports of restored libido and healthy sexual responses.

Mary may have been "only" 33, but her testosterone level was *less than* 10 ng/dl, with an estradiol of only 40 pg/ml on day 3 of her cycle. Her low hormone levels, especially for her age, correspond exactly with her descriptions of the changes and problems she was having.

Yet Mary also had a difficult time getting help. She told me that when she asked her primary physician what could be causing her loss of interest in sex, his reply (based only on her *age*) was, "*Well, I guess you'll need some marital therapy. It must be a problem in your relationship.*"

Mary then asked about having her hormones tested. She said her doctor told her, "*There's no way to do that, and it doesn't mean anything anyway.*"

When she had her consultation with me, an integral part of my evaluation was to measure the blood levels of testosterone. She had been willing to consider marital therapy, but not until someone had at least checked the *hormonal* aspects. Based on her insight, self-awareness and research, she honestly felt that her problem was more likely a *physical* change, since she sincerely felt her martial relationship was very good. She loved her husband very much, they weren't having any unusual stresses, and she had always enjoyed sex so much.

Consider:

Female sexual dysfunction (FSD) is age-related, progressive and highly prevalent.

It is true that there is no real agreement among specialists as to an "optimal" range for testosterone for women to feel their best and have a healthy sex drive. So?

Experts didn't agree on optimal cholesterol levels either for most of my medical career. Only very recently, after much research, have nationally accepted cholesterol guidelines been recommended. Yet, for twenty-five years, I have practiced medicine checking cholesterol levels and making clinical judgments for individuals, taking into account their entire picture and health risks.

We can do the same with testosterone.

It is also true that measuring testosterone is more difficult in women than men because our testosterone levels are so much lower. Current assays for testosterone don't give as reliable a reading in the low ranges a woman's body produces. But what we *do have* for testosterone blood tests is still a lot *better than doing nothing* to check this critical hormone!

After working with women on these issues for over twenty years, I have found that an optimal testosterone range for women appears to be between 40—60 ng/dl (or 400—600 pg/ml). That's the range on blood tests that best corresponds with my patients telling me they feel "back to my old spark" or "I finally *want* to have sex again."

Of course, the range of what is "normal" for an individual woman can vary quite a bit within, or even below, this range, but most of my patients describe feeling what *they* consider their "normal" sex drive and interest in sex if blood levels are somewhere between 40-60 ng/dl about four hours after an oral or cream dose of testosterone.

My patients who still have testosterone levels lower than 40 ng/dl four hours after taking it typically report that their sexual interest hasn't returned.

If the testosterone levels are too much higher than 60 ng/dl, they often report feeling sexual urges that are too intense or unpleasant or intrusive. At higher testosterone levels, they also tell me they feel more irritable, edgy, tense, aggressive, and don't sleep as restfully. Sometimes, women tell me they know the testosterone is too much because they are troubled by aggressive, violent, frightening dreams. This is especially true if another doctor has told them to take testosterone at night. Women's testosterone normally *peaks in the morning,* and declines in the evening.

To give you a sense of perspective, men's testosterone levels normally run about 500-1200 ng/dl. Most men don't experience a loss of libido until testosterone drops down to around 500 or less, although again, this may vary slightly depending on what is "normal" for a given man. Because women's optimal ranges for testosterone are so much lower and narrower, women are more sensitive to a much smaller change: what appears to be only a slight drop of 10-15 ng/dl *can make an enormous difference* in whether a woman will feel her usual sexual spark.

To clarify the numbers I have given above: you may find different books quoting ranges for testosterone that will seem quite different from those I have given. The differences occur because laboratories may use different units of measure.

Throughout my book, I am using *nanograms* per deciliter (ng/dl) in the testosterone ranges because that is the

Attention:

FSD may affect up to 43% of pre-menopausal women and 60% of sexually active post-menopausal women.

unit of measure used more commonly by labs in the U.S. Ranges reported in other units can appear quite different until the proper conversion is made. Take a look, though, at what the level of testosterone would be for women if we use the same units for testosterone that we used for estradiol.

Estradiol is measured in **pg/ml**: 200 pg/ml is typical of about Day 20

Testosterone level of 40-60 **ng/dl** converts to **400-600 pg/ml.** That is about *2-3 times the amount of the estradiol* peak the second half of a typical menstrual cycle.

The following chart shows how all these hormones relate to one another, once they are all expressed in the same units of measure.

I think this comparison really puts in perspective just how much *more testosterone* than estrogen a woman makes during her reproductive years, not to mention the other androgens our bodies make. Clearly, androgens are an important group of compounds for women!

Mean Ovarian Hormone Levels in Women Not Taking Hormones
(all converted to pg/ml)

	Fertile, 20s-30s (average across menstrual cycle)	Natural menopause (no HRT)	Surgical menopause (no HRT)
Estradiol	100-150	10-15	10
Testosterone	400-600	290	110
Androstenedione	1900-2000	1000	700
DHEA	4000-5000	2000	1800
DHEA-S	3,000,000	1,000,000	1,000,000

(adapted from: Simpson E., Androgens in Women, Fertil Steril 2002, Lobo R. Treatment of Postmenopausal Women, Boston: Lippincott, 1999)

Women's Sexual Response: Just What is "Normal"

One of the most common problems I encounter in my medical practice is *a lack of knowledge* about the human sexual response in men and women. Popular movies and magazines often portray romanticized or exaggerated sexual activities and perpetuate unrealistic performance expectations for what is "normal." There are also many myths about what's "normal" sexual response, especially for women. They need to be put to rest because they perpetuate a loss of self-confidence and positive self image that are so important to a healthy sexuality. What are some of these myths? Take a look at the following chart, and see if these reflect some of your own thinking.

From Dr. Ruth:

"Be realistic. Even with loving couples, sexual appetite waxes and wanes."

TEN COMMON Sexual Myths

#1:   Loss of sexual desire is due to deep-seated psychological conflicts

#2:   Being sexually active is a sign of emotional health.

#3:   Normal couples have sex on average twice a week.

#4:   Men are supposed to have higher sex drives than women

#5:   Women should have vaginal orgasm with intercourse rather than orgasm from clitoral stimulation

#6:   Vaginal orgasms during intercourse indicate a more "mature" sexual response than clitoral orgasm

#7:   Women are supposed to have multiple orgasms with intercourse

#8:   Orgasm during pregnancy can cause a miscarriage

#9:   Loss of interest in sex means you don't love your partner

#10: Psychological factors cause more sexual problems than do hormone changes as women get older.

All of the above statements are false.

Let's look at a few facts to dispel some of these outmoded ideas.

FACT: Many women find great emotional satisfaction from sex, but that doesn't mean everyone has to be sexually active to be "emotionally healthy." And likewise, as you can see from my patients' quotes at the beginning of this chapter, a lack of sexual desire is not always an indicator of deep psychological problems.

Wisdom:

It's quality over quantity.

FACT: There are marked individual differences in sex drive. Some men have low sex drive that is normal for them, and some women have a very high sex drive that is also perfectly normal. Most of us lie somewhere in between, and our sex drive changes greatly at various stages of our lives, and during times of increased stress and life demands.

FACT: There's no one right magic number for frequency of sex. Are you more emotionally stable if you have sex more often? Less often? Some couples have sex once a week, some have sex almost daily, and others have sex once or twice a year. The whole range of frequency is considered "normal," depending upon what is mutually satisfying for each couple. No one should have to live up to an arbitrary standard of "normal" frequency for sex. Pay attention to what feels right for you in your relationship. If you both are happy with where you are, then that's "normal" for you. If either or both of you is unhappy, that's the time to work on finding out what's out-of-kilter and begin making positive changes.

FACT: There is absolutely no scientific basis to the theory that "vaginal" orgasms are more "mature" than "clitoral" orgasms. This theory is still widely believed, based on the authority of none other than Dr. Sigmund Freud, famous psychoanalyst. This idea was based on Freud's theory that as women matured psychologically, they were able to reach orgasm from stimulation by the thrusting of the penis in the vagina. Freud believed that women who could only achieve orgasm with direct stimulation of the clitoris were not as psychologically mature, and needed intensive psychoanalysis to resolve unconscious conflicts that prevented them from reaching vaginal orgasm. Over the years of my clinical practice, I have seen a lot of damage caused by this outmoded theory, with many women feeling a sense of shame and inadequacy because they didn't reach orgasm with vaginal penetration.

FACT: Our understanding of the physiology of women's sexual response has progressed significantly since Freud's time. We now know that it doesn't matter which way a woman reaches orgasm—both are equal ways of achieving the pleasurable sensations that go with release of sexual tension from arousal.

FACT: Drs. Perry and Whipple demonstrated in a 1981 study that two different nerve pathways in the pelvis carry sexual stimulation messages and orgasm can be produced with stimulation of either pathway. Clitoral *or* vaginal stimulation can trigger orgasm via the *pudendal* nerve, while cervical *or* vaginal stimulation can trigger orgasm via the *pelvic* nerve. This means that a number of sensory nerve bundles can influence orgasm with stimulation of different areas in the pelvis. For women who have had their cervix removed with a hysterectomy, it means there is still an intact vaginal-clitoral nerve pathway to orgasm. For women who are making the decision about whether to *keep* the cervix when facing a hysterectomy, knowledge of these nerve pathways may tip the balance toward keeping the cervix and having a *supracervical hysterectomy.*

FACT: Other research has found that the *rhythm* of sexual stimulation to the clitoris and vagina, along with optimal hormone levels, may be more critical for orgasm than whether stimulation is clitoral or vaginal or both.

Enjoy!

It doesn't matter which road you take, getting there is half the fun... and the final destination is the same.

The bottom line? Don't feel that you are somehow less of a woman because you only reach orgasm one way.

FACT: It's not just loss of ovarian hormones that can cause loss of sexual desire. There are many other endocrine changes, medical disorders, and medications that can sap your libido. A good example of this is something as common as birth control pills, as you saw with Laurie at the beginning of the chapter. Oral birth control pills can increase SHBG and lower free testosterone, leading to loss of sex drive. High progestin pills, such as Laurie was given, reduce sex drive and sexual responsiveness even further by also blocking the testosterone receptors.

Wisdom:

The way we view ourselves affects our sexuality.

FACT: Loss of sex drive, and reduced ability to have an orgasm, can occur when you take antidepressants, or sleeping pills, or "mood-stabilizer" medicines, or beta blockers, and many other common OTC and Rx medications.

FACT: Medical illnesses, like early diabetes, even if not yet diagnosed, can lead to low sex drive and reduced nerve sensitivity that makes it harder to reach orgasm. These are just a few of many physical causes of low sex drive. I will explore others in later chapters and teach you what you can to do overcome them.

Changes As We Age: Effects on Our Hormones of Desire and Arousal

Our entire body undergoes many different physical and psychological changes as we get older. It shouldn't come a surprise that there are major changes affecting sexual function as well.

Some changes as we age are caused by the decline in the "sex hormones" from the ovaries; some are caused by other hormone and metabolic factors. Some are the result of our changing view of ourselves, other changes in sexual function happen because of life stress and changes in our relationship. It is a complex tapestry of many interwoven dimensions of our lives. All are important to take into account.

The bottom line is, we can't ignore the basic facts of biology: hormones produced by the ovaries play critical roles in our entire sexual response—from activating the brain's "sexual circuits" to regulating pelvic blood flow, nerve sensitivity, vaginal lubrication and muscle tone that are all needed in a healthy sexual response.

Ovarian hormones, primarily estradiol and testosterone, are our "mood elevating" hormones as well. Both estradiol and testosterone contribute dramatically to positive, vibrant, upbeat moods and our sense of psychological well-being. Without them, we can feel flat, blue, blah, and disinterested...often, with low levels of both, women describe feeling a lack motivation to do much of anything, especially sex!

There are many good books about the psychological issues that affect us as we age. It is beyond the focus of this book to go into depth on these dimensions. My primary goal here is to explain how your "sex hormones" play such important roles in your sexual function. I want to help you understand how the loss of optimal levels of testosterone and estradiol have profound effects on all aspects of your ability to be interested in sex, and your ability to respond to sexual stimulation.

I feel it is crucial to understand the physical endocrine changes that are taking place because they have such a major impact on all the other dimensions of our sexual life and physical-emotional well-being. I explain these hormone effects in the sections that follow, and I summarized the most important physical and psychological consequences of losing testosterone and estradiol in the charts that follow.

Dr. VLIET'S GUIDE to MIND-BODY Changes Affecting Women's Sexuality As We Age

PHYSICAL CHANGES:
(primarily caused by hormone decline)

- ↑ FSH, LH
- ↓ estradiol
- ↓ testosterone
- ↓ androstenedione
- ↓ DHEA, and DHEA-S
- ↓ vaginal thickness and elasticity
- ↓ vaginal lubrication
- ↓ vaginal blood flow
- ↑ vaginal pH (more alkaline)
- ↓ size of cervix, uterus, ovaries
- ↓ decreased breast/nipple sensitivity
- ↓ decreased vaginal muscle tone and strength
- ↓ intensity of vaginal and uterine muscle contractions during orgasm
- ↓ sensitivity of nerve endings (clitoris, cervix, nipples)

(Note: progesterone also declines, but low levels have not been shown to have adverse effect on women's sexual response)

PSYCHOLOGICAL CHANGES:
(mediated by hormone decline, life stress, relationship changes, medications, other factors)

- ↓ sexual desire
- ↓ sexual fantasies, thoughts
- ↓ sexual receptivity (to touch, etc.)
- ↓ masturbation frequency
- ↓ mood
- ↓ motivation
- ↓ energy level
- ↓ satisfaction with body
- ↑ sexual avoidance

©Elizabeth Lee Vliet, MD 2005

Androgens as Sexual "Activators"

Think of testosterone, along with our other androgens, as "activators" at the brain centers that stimulate sexual desire. Testosterone helps us initiate sex; it acts much like using a match to start a fire. Because of this, testosterone is called the hormone of desire in both men and women.

Just as it's hard to light a fire with a wet match, it's hard to light the sexual fires in the brain if your testosterone tank is close to empty. These brain pathways need adequate testosterone, *and* adequate estradiol, for women to be able to initiate and respond optimally to sexual activity.

Multiple clinical trials and other research studies from many different countries have found consistent results: *low* testosterone levels in women leads to loss of sexual thoughts and fantasies, loss of sexual content in dreams, diminished desire for sex and even sexual avoidance. When our testosterone is too low, we often experience a lack of "drive" in other ways too, not just sex drive. We lose motivation to do things we once enjoyed. We feel blah. We don't have as much energy, or as a number of women have said to me, "My get-up-and-go has got-up-and-gone!"

Conversely, when testosterone levels are in an optimal range, studies consistently show that women are more likely to think about, desire, and initiate sexual activity. Women describe enhanced sexual gratification, they have more desire to masturbate, and they report more sexual thoughts, fantasies, and dreams. In short, a vibrant, healthy, lusty sexual life becomes possible with our biological testosterone "activator" hormone intact to light the fire.

At the other extreme, women with *excess* testosterone typically describe having unpleasant, intrusive increases in sex drive. Patients have said "I feel like I have this sensation in my clitoris all the time that I have to relieve with masturbation, but then it comes right back."

Wisdom:

Optimal testosterone levels lead to more sexual fantasies and thoughts.

One woman in her forties, who had been given a high dose testosterone cream by a compounding pharmacist, said "This constant urge to have sex is driving me nuts. Now I know what my 17-year-old son must have been going though with his surging hormones! I don't like this at all!"

At even higher levels, such as doses used by body-builders abusing testosterone and other anabolic steroids to lose fat and build muscle, women lose breast tissue, have excess facial hair, and *both* men and women develop toxic behavioral effects such as: extreme irritability, volatile/explosive moods, aggressiveness or assaultiveness. Interestingly, at such high doses of androgens, women bodybuilders estradiol is too suppressed and they may actually have low libido, vaginal dryness, painful sex and problems reaching orgasm.

It Takes to Two to Tango—The Sexual Dance of Estradiol and Testosterone

From my clinical evaluations of women over the years, it has become clear to me that for us to have a healthy libido, adequate vaginal lubrication and ability to reach orgasm, we need an optimal level of both estradiol and testosterone, in the right balance. Excess or deficit or one or the other can lead to problems with sexual function.

My observations and study of hormone levels in patients fits with findings from neuroendocrine research that suggests for testosterone to activate brain receptors, there needs to be "priming" of those androgen receptors by estrogen, in particular, estradiol. If estradiol is too low, I find that even really high levels of androgens don't usually lead to *high sex drive* in women.

Estradiol plays a crucial role in women being able to have healthy vaginal lubrication with sexual stimulation. Women whose estradiol levels are quite low often have severe problems with vaginal dryness, and even may have vulvar pain (vulvodynia). Even if these women have adequate testosterone, they tell me that their interest in sex has waned because of the dryness and pain. On the other hand, I have seen women with high levels of estradiol and good vaginal lubrication who had low testosterone and had little interest in sex.

Surprise:

Men and women have different sexual response patterns

Estradiol, along with testosterone, also helps to stimulate more blood flow to the pelvis and vagina and to enhance sensitivity of clitoral and cervical nerve endings to sexual stimulation. Increased blood flow, called *vasocongestion,* intensifies our arousal and contributes to what we experience as "sexual tension" during foreplay. After reaching orgasm, vasocongestion then resolves, and we feel a relief of the pelvic sexual tension.

Progesterone and progestins are inhibitors of sexual arousal at brain centers regulating sexual response. High levels of prolactin, a pituitary hormone that regulates milk production for nursing, also causes central nervous system inhibition of sexual drive and arousal. Low levels of thyroid hormones have a similar effect to inhibit brain centers involved in desire and arousal.

Understanding A Woman's Sexual Response: New Insights

In the 1960s, Dr. William Masters and Virginia Johnson pioneered the study of male and female sexual response, and developed a model describing a linear progression from Arousal/excitement to Plateau to Orgasm and then Resolution as I illustrated in the following chart. Their model was primarily focused on the physical genital and breast responses to sexual stimuli. Their work was ground-breaking at the time, and opened the door to better understanding of the physical aspects of sexual arousal with their detailed descriptions of body changes in men and women at each stage. Masters and Johnson, however, assumed that men and women had similar patterns of responding to sexual stimuli, although they recognized that women generally had a longer arousal and plateau phase than men did.

Impact Of Hormone Loss On Women's Physical Sexual Responsiveness By Master's And Johnson Stages

Excitement/Arousal Phase:

- slowed response, takes longer to become aroused
- reduced blood flow to vagina/pelvis leads to decreased ability to become aroused
- reduced vaginal lubrication (increases pain)
- decreased breast engorgement
- reduced nipple sensitivity
- diminished clitoral sensitivity

Plateau Phase:

- reduced elevation of uterus during arousal
- reduced flattening and separation of labia
- diminished increase in clitoral size (due to reduced blood flow to pelvis)

Orgasm Phase:

- more stimulation needed to reach orgasm
- orgasm shorter in duration, less intense
- uterine and vaginal muscle contractions less intense, and do not last as long.
- Uterine contractions may be painful for some women (e.g. if large fibroids are present)

Resolution Phase:

- shorter duration of pleasurable effects from arousal
- more rapid return to prestimulation level
- clitorial and breast engorgement quickly subsides
- more difficult to have multiple orgasms

©Elizabeth Lee Vliet, MD 1995-2005

Later, in the 1970s, Dr. Helen Singer Kaplan refined the Masters and Johnson model, and described the phases of sexual response as Desire, Arousal, Orgasm, and Resolution. Again, Dr. Kaplan viewed the response patterns to be similar for men and women, and her model had the same linear progression from one stage to the next.

None of these earlier models adequately addressed other factors that may motivate women to want sex, such as desire for emotional intimacy. Nor did these earlier models address the concept of *satisfaction,* so important in human beings. One can be emotionally and physically satisfied with a sexual experience even when there is no orgasm. Satisfaction goes beyond just having intercourse to reach orgasm, and considers the physical, emotional, and spiritual pleasure from the entire erotic encounter between two people.

As we began to study women's sexual responses in more depth, however, it became clear that many women, did not progress step-wise through this sequence of sexual stages. This was especially true for older women and women in long-standing, stable relationships, who were more likely to engage in sex as an expression of intimacy and love for their partner, whether or not they *first* had the desire, or were even aroused themselves. As an outgrowth of these new understandings, Dr. Rosemary Basson proposed a new model, called the Intimacy-based model.

Dr. Basson's model is on the following page. I amplified her model with aspects that I think are important based on my clinical experience. I think this helps to see the many different dimensions that affect women's receptivity to having sex and their ability to respond fully, from the physical/biological/hormonal, to psychological, situational, and even spiritual aspects of our being. It is also important to keep in mind that each one of these dimensions affects the others, in a circular and even criss-cross fashion.

For example, women with vaginal dryness causing pain with intercourse (*dyspareunia*) will often experience loss

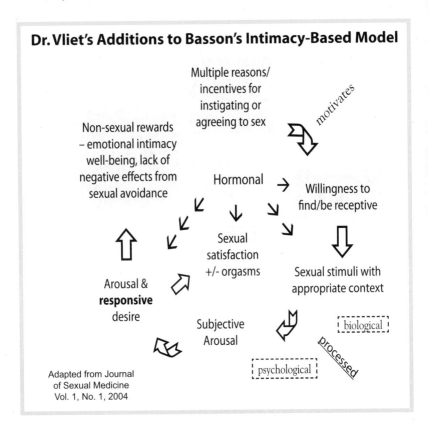

Dr. Vliet's Additions to Basson's Intimacy-Based Model

Multiple reasons/ incentives for instigating or agreeing to sex

motivates

Non-sexual rewards – emotional intimacy well-being, lack of negative effects from sexual avoidance

Hormonal

Willingness to find/be receptive

Sexual satisfaction +/- orgasms

Arousal & **responsive** desire

Sexual stimuli with appropriate context

Subjective Arousal

biological

processed

psychological

Adapted from Journal of Sexual Medicine Vol. 1, No. 1, 2004

of desire from fear of more pain, and may have arousal difficulty because fear and pain signals interfere with the relaxation needed to become aroused. A *physical* problem triggers a *psychological* response that in turn causes more *physical* limitations or pain. Pain itself triggers more suppression of estradiol and testosterone, causing more vaginal dryness, and then more pain. You can see how it can become a vicious cycle.

Women who have been raped or otherwise traumatized sexually may have memories that trigger involuntary vaginal muscle contractions, and make penetration difficult or impossible even when they love their partner and no longer consciously feel fearful. They may not even realize these contractions of the vaginal muscle are happening. Again, pain limits ability to respond sexually, potentially triggering many different psychological and relationship problems. In evaluating women with these problems, it is important to consider all of these dimensions, and look at the variety of therapeutic modalities available to help.

Varieties of Women's Sexual Dysfunction

What is meant by "sexual dysfunction"? Given the complexity of our sexual responses as humans, that has been a challenging question for many years. Old concepts of "fridgity" in women and "impotence" in men have finally given way to a more systematic way of classifying sexual problems that also helps us focus on the types of treatment needed. Newer ways of thinking about sexual problems have also gotten away from the earlier focus on mental/psychological aspects to look more closely at the biological causes of these problems.

The World Health Organization describes sexual dysfunction as *"the various ways in which an individual is unable to participate in a sexual relationship as he or she would wish."*

The American Psychiatric Association defines sexual dysfunction as *"disturbances in sexual desire and in the psychophysiological changes that characterize the sexual response cycle and cause marked distress and interpersonal difficulty."*

The degree to which you feel distress about a particular aspect of your sexual functioning is a key issue that makes the *problem* a *dysfunction.* For example, low sex drive in itself isn't a "disorder." Some people are perfectly happy having low sex drive. If you aren't feeling at all distressed by loss of sexual desire, then it doesn't rise to the level of being a "disorder." If it is causing personal or relationship *distress,* however, then it is a dysfunction worthy of careful evaluation and treatment.

We now classify female sexual dysfunction (FSD) into the following groups, based on the sexual response phases: *desire* (libido), *arousal* (excitement), and *orgasm.* Keep in mind, it isn't an either—or situation. Each type of sexual problem can have a combination of causes, and many women may have more than one type of problem, as my patient's story at the end of this chapter illustrates.

Female Sexual Dysfunction (FSD) Classification And Definitions:

Disorders of Sexual Desire

1. **Hypoactive Sexual Desire Disorder (HSDD)**—*Persistent deficiency or absence of sexual thoughts, fantasies, and/or receptivity to sexual activity that causes personal distress.*

2. **Sexual Aversion Disorder**—*Persistent or recurrent avoidance of sexual activity that causes personal distress.*

Disorders of Sexual Arousal

1. **Difficulty with lubrication**—*reduced or absent vaginal secretions in response to sexual stimulation*

2. **Diminished clitoral/labial sensation**—*reduced or absent sensory response to sexual stimulation*

3. **Diminished engorgement**—*reduced pelvic vasocongestion (blood flow) response to sexual stimulation*

4. Inadequate vaginal muscle relaxation

Orgasmic Disorders

1. **Primary**—one has never achieved orgasm

2. **Secondary**—one has been able to have orgasms in the past and is no longer able to.

Sexual Pain Disorders

1. **Vaginismus**—*involuntary muscle contractions of the muscles of the outer portion of the vagina that causes significant pain with attempted penetration*

2. **Dyspareunia**—*persistent or recurrent vaginal and/or vulvar pain with sexual intercourse*

3. **Noncoital sexual pain**—*pain that occurs in the genital area other than with intercourse.*

Source: International Consensus Development Conference on FSD Guidelines, J. of Urology, 2000.

Gay is a 47-year-old married woman referred to me by her therapist because of her difficulties with painful sex, vaginal dryness and menopausal symptoms. At her consult recently, Gay said:

> "My problems began in my early forties when I started having cyclic episodes of vaginal dryness and painful intercourse. Then it would go away for a few weeks, but it would always come back. After a while I finally realized there was a pattern to it. It seemed to always happen right before my period started, then it would get better a few days after my period ended. My family doctor acted like he thought the problems were all in my head. I began to wonder if there was some hormonal problem because it always happened right around my period. Finally my family doctor let me try some estrogen vaginal cream and that helped. But my OBGyn didn't want me to use any hormones, so I stopped the cream.
>
> After my periods stopped when I was 46, the pain with sex got worse and worse. I was so dry, having sex felt like I was being scrubbed inside with sand paper. It also felt like my vagina was narrowing. When we would try to have sex, it felt like my husband hit something hard and couldn't go in any further, like he was hitting something that was on the part of my vagina that's against my rectum. Sometimes he could get past that ridge and we could have sex but it was never comfortable. Besides not being able to lubricate, I have this burning pain after sex. It has gotten so bad that my husband is afraid to try sex because he doesn't want to hurt me."

I kept thinking it had to be something physical, so I saw my Gyn for an exam. That really hurt, but all he said was my vaginal wall looked like Arnold Schwarzenegger's muscles. I didn't know what he meant by that, and he didn't explain it. He didn't really suggest any treatment except he said I needed to see a sex therapist. His response always seemed to revert to it's in my head, and there's nothing *physically wrong. He said there's no way to check hormones. The therapist I have seen off and on for stress management really thinks there is something more to it, and he suggested I see you. He has worked with me on some relationship issues and that's been a big help, but he wanted someone to check the medical and hormonal aspects. He doesn't think it is just a psychological issue the way my Gyn seems to."*

In addition to the problems with painful intercourse and vaginal dryness, Gay described a number of other symptoms that really bothered her: dry eyes to the point that she couldn't wear her contacts any more, profound tiredness that made it hard for her to get through her day at work, almost daily dull headaches, restless sleep, trouble concentrating at work and being more forgetful about tasks she needed to do. She was too tired to exercise like she had been accustomed to doing regularly. She said:

"I don't feel like myself any more. I've always been so successful at work, had no trouble multi-tasking and keeping up with the demands of a very busy office. Now I feel like I am losing it. I don't have any get up and go, I don't have any libido and I feel like I have this diminished sensation all over my body, not just sexually."

Her examination and laboratory studies helped provide an explanation for her puzzling cluster of problems. Her estradiol was extremely low at 9 pg/ml, and her menopausal level of FSH at 67 reflected her low estradiol. Her total testosterone was only 14 ng/dl, with a free testosterone of 2 pg/ml, both also very low. Her thyroid, adrenal, cholesterol and metabolic studies were excellent, indicating no problems in these areas of her health.

Her physical examination was normal except for one significant finding: a sustained contraction of the outer vaginal muscles. She was not even aware she was contracting these muscles, but the involuntary spasm created such a tight ring at the vaginal opening that it prevented my using even the smallest speculum to fully examine the inside of the vagina. Her vaginal opening was so constricted by the tight muscles that it barely allowed insertion of a lubricated, gloved finger, and even that was uncomfortable for her.

I explained that the medical term for her condition is *vaginismus*, a sustained contraction of the outer vaginal muscles that makes penetration difficult and painful. During the exam, I gently pressed on the muscle ring to show her where it was, and she said with some relief, *"That's the hard area I feel when my husband tries to enter, that's what felt like a ridge that he couldn't get past."* I explained how the low estradiol causes vaginal dryness and pain, and then a reflex muscle contraction begins to occur in anticipation of more pain. Then the muscle tightness makes it painful for penetration, and more pain causes more tensing of the muscles. It's a vicious cycle, and we needed to tackle the problem several ways.

In addition, her low estradiol and low testosterone also contributed to her marked fatigue, low libido, headaches, dry eyes, and difficulty concentrating. Low estradiol also was a major culprit in her restless, fragmented sleep. The vaginal dryness, as well as her lack of lubrication during sex, was primarily caused by her low estrogen.

I talked with her about an integrated approach to treatment:

- continuing with her therapist, as a couple, to help her husband understand all of these findings and how he could help,

- a series of exercises to teach her how to relax the vaginal muscles,

- relaxation and visual imagery training to help her overcome her fear of pain that contributed to the muscle tension

- restoring her hormone levels to more optimal ranges with bioidentical estradiol lotion (Estrasorb), bioidentical testosterone in a sustained release capsule, and a compounded hypoallergenic estradiol vaginal cream free of irritating preservatives to avoid aggravating the sensitive vaginal tissue.

Gay described feeling a sense of relief and validation now that she understood the different physical, hormonal, and psychological factors that were all contributing to her loss of desire for sex and the pain she had been having whenever she and her husband attempted to have sex. She was pleased to find out that she had been right: her low hormone levels were playing a significant role in her problems, and more importantly, there was something she could do about it.

Gay's story illustrates the importance of taking a comprehensive view of women's sexual problems, since there can be several different types that need to be addressed, and a number of causes. Certainly the low estradiol and testosterone were critical issues that had been overlooked by previous physicians, but she also needed to understand the physical problems of vaginal dryness and vaginismus. She needed to know how pain from these physical problems set up a psychological vicious cycle of anticipatory anxiety from fear of pain, which created more stress that further suppressed her estradiol and testosterone, and caused more pain. Her feelings of inadequacy about sex further compounded the loss of desire triggered by low hormone levels.

She was perfectly happy to work with a therapist on these psychological dimensions now that she better understand how all the pieces of the puzzle fit together. What had bothered her, she said, however, was continually being referred to a therapist before anyone had evaluated the hormone and physical aspects that she had been asking about for so long.

Restoring Your Sexual Vitality

Being able to enjoy sex, and have a healthy, vital sexual response is an important dimension of our well-being, whether we are with a partner or during self-pleasuring. It is long overdue for medicine to focus on ways of helping women overcome the many different types of sexual problems, but we are slowly making headway. Women's loss of sexual responsiveness causes distress and suffering for many. It is no less important than loss of sexual function is for men.

Enjoyment of our sexuality certainly doesn't *have* to decline as women approach menopause and hormones wane. There are many avenues for keep your sexual interest and vitality alive and well. Some of these you control, as I will discuss in Chapter 10, and some options are medications and hormones as I have described in this chapter for you to explore with your physician.

Although many women may be uncomfortable talking about these problems with physicians, it's important to bring up your concerns. There are many new medical techniques and treatments available, and you need to be proactive about discussing your concerns with your health professionals.

A variety of educational programs in recent years have encouraged physicians and other health professionals to include questions about sexual health as part of the usual health histories. Even if your doctor doesn't bring up these issues, he or she should be receptive to your opening the discussion.

Before you visit your doctor, you may find it helpful to explore your feelings about your sexuality in the Self-Test questionnaire in Chapter 10: "How's My Sexuality?" I wrote this many years ago to help my patients think about what concerns they had, and organize their thoughts prior to an office appointment. Jot down whatever comes to mind about each of these questions. This will give you a list of topics to help you focus your questions in the time you have with your doctor. If you find that you have more questions and concerns than you realized, you may want to seek a specialist in this field.

In this chapter and Chapter 10, I have been able to review only the highlights of aspects important in enhancing your sexual vitality. There are many books totally devoted to this subject, as I listed in the Resources section of the Appendix. These will give you additional information and ideas for rekindling the sexual fires. I particularly recommend Dr. Miriam Stoppard's classic book, *The Magic of Sex*, as an outstanding comprehensive, beautifully illustrated and sensitively written guide for sexual enjoyment for men and women.

Don't let your questions and concerns about the physical role of hormones be overlooked, dismissed, and discounted. Don't just start an antidepressant if you feel other issues have not been adequately evaluated. If your physician doesn't seem interested or knowledgeable in these areas, then find one who is.

Remember too that if you want zesty sex life, it is important to feel good about yourself and your body. Avoid buying into the images that bombard us about what a "perfect" body is supposed to look like. Don't focus on what's "wrong" with your body rather than what is "right" about it. There is no "perfect" body! Focus on boosting your self-confidence by working to develop a *healthy* body. Pay attention to getting proper evaluation of potential physical or medical causes of sexual problems. Push for what you need to have done to get your questions answered.

Don't just suffer silently. Know that help is available and that you deserve to enjoy sex, whatever your age!

Chapter 4

Testosterone Effects Throughout The Body

Throughout a woman's life, testosterone has important functions in maintaining energy, strength and stamina. It is a major metabolic fuel that helps run our engines—without it, we'd be like a car without gas. With an empty gas tank, you could push your car and make it move, but it certainly wouldn't be an efficient way to use a car for transportation!

Likewise, without enough testosterone to fuel our body engines and help us feel energetic, we literally are having to "push" the body through our days—feeling tired, run-down, blah, and out of steam. Loss of the critical metabolic hormone testosterone is one of the frequently unrecognized factors in the midlife problem of "chronic fatigue," especially when it is accompanied by low levels of it's crucial metabolic partner, estradiol.

Many women have multiple medical evaluations and spend hundreds or thousands of dollars on tests and therapies to diagnose and treat "chronic fatigue" (CFS) and *never have a blood level test for testosterone or estradiol.*

Testosterone also plays an enormous role in building and repairing healthy muscle tissue. That is why it is called an anabolic hormone, because it stimulates the building of muscle and bone, our lean body mass, and uses our fat stores for the fuel to make lean tissue. Using our fat stores to **build** more muscle means our body composition improves, and we have a lower percent of body fat, even if the scale doesn't show changes in pounds. While we don't become "muscle bound" or develop

Fact:

Testosterone is a major metabolic fuel. Make sure your tank isn't on empty!

the huge muscles that men do, women still need optimal testosterone to maintain muscle mass. Without it, we lose muscle and become flabby and fatter as we age.

At menopause when our ovaries are no longer our primary hormone-producing factories, women lose both estradiol and testosterone, and this causes us to lose muscle and bone faster than men because we experience a more dramatic and sudden loss of testosterone. Men's testosterone falls much more slowly, over many years, so they lose muscle mass and bone more gradually, and later in life.

Muscles!

The more muscle you have, the more calories you burn.

Work those muscles!

And don't forget, our muscle tissue is that wonderful "fat burning," machinery. Muscle burns more calories per minute every minute of every day than any other tissue in our body. The more muscle you have, the more calories you burn, even when you are not exercising.

Fat tissue is more sluggish, and burns far fewer calories per minute than muscle tissue does. Loss of muscle slows our metabolic rate. Our body composition shifts toward more fat.

Less muscles = less calories burned = more flabby fat, year by year.

Lower testosterone levels also mean less ability to *build* muscle, *even if* you are exercising several times a week. Your muscles simply don't respond to exercise as well if you don't have optimal testosterone and estradiol levels. So as you get older, you need adequate testosterone to keep your metabolic engines revved up and your muscles strong.

Testosterone has to be balanced with the right amount of estradiol or you will start packing on pounds around your middle. When estradiol declines, it results in a dominance of androgens, made in the adrenal glands and fat tissue, that in turn begin to produce those unsightly upper body fat deposits…you know, that dangling underarm fat, and the fat pads that feel like breasts growing out your side!

The androgen excess makes our bodies morph from the young woman's pear-shape to the health-risky apple shape that looks a lot like the "beer belly" in older men. The hormone imbalances and resulting apple shape lead to additional unwanted metabolic changes: increasing blood pressure, increasing total cholesterol, and decreasing HDL ("good") cholesterol, along with increasing LDL ("bad") cholesterol, and higher insulin and cortisol. All of these changes contribute to the increasing risks of heart disease, hypertension, and diabetes in women as they get older.

At first, doctors blamed testosterone for these negative effects on the cholesterol ratio and insulin response. Newer studies have shown, however, that testosterone actually helps improve insulin sensitivity, and helps maintain the normal mechanisms involved in dilating blood vessels to help lower blood pressure, *only if* it is given with the right balance of estradiol.

If given *alone* to women, testosterone and DHEA act to promote build up artery-clogging plaque (atherosclerosis). If the androgens are *given with* estradiol, however, they have the opposite effect on the arterial wall and actually help prevent build-up of plaque in the arteries.

Testosterone also plays a key role along with estradiol to help *build bone* and prevent osteoporosis. Multiple studies worldwide have shown the bone-building effects of testosterone in women of different ethnic groups. Women have increased bone breakdown as estrogen declines leading up to menopause, so your level of testosterone becomes even more crucial in maintaining bone density when your estradiol is low as well. I find that my patients see the most improvement in reversing bone loss and building healthy new bone when they take an appropriate amount of estradiol *and* restore testosterone to optimal levels, too.

There is a myth perpetrated by the sellers of OTC hormone and wild yam creams that progesterone in these creams helps build bone and muscle and lose fat by giving the body the building blocks to make more testosterone and estrogen from progesterone as a precursor. If you are menopausal, either surgically or naturally, this is false.

The process of progesterone being converted to testosterone and then estradiol requires enzymes and reactions

New Findings:

Testosterone in balance with E2, can help *lower* blood pressure and help *build* bone.

that take place in *functioning* ovaries. If you are menopausal or have had a hysterectomy or tubal ligation or chemotherapy that damages the ovaries, then you don't have the working pathways to properly convert progesterone to testosterone and estradiol. You end up having a load of progesterone that simply makes you fatter by blocking the activity of what estradiol and testosterone you have left.

Marta Keeps Riding

Marta is a 47-year-old massage therapist who had been an avid runner and cyclist most of her adult life. In her late thirties and early forties, she had even won two national titles in tandem biking. She had noticed a gradual but significant decrease in her stamina and energy on the rides over the past three years, and was having more problems with tendonitis that kept her from being able to run as much as she usually did.

Wisdom:

Changes in menstrual flow patterns can be a clue to hormone imbalances.

She was also losing hair, and noticed that she was getting much "thicker" around her waist. She had gained about 36 pounds over the last three years, and nothing she did with diet or all her exercise seemed to bring back her waistline or help lose this excess weight.

She also began to notice that she didn't have the same strength in her hands to do massage therapy as she always had, and had recently started having achey joints in her arms and hands and hips that made it even harder to work. She felt sluggish and tired, not at all like her usual energetic self!

Her family doctor told her she was probably just depressed, and recommended an antidepressant. She felt awful on that, gained even more weight, and didn't notice any improvement in her energy level or strength.

She was still menstruating regularly, but her periods had become much lighter and the flow only lasted a day or two now instead of the usual four or five days she used to have. She thought that was strange, and asked to have her hormones checked, but even her *female* GYN would not agree to do this. She said, "My Gynecologist just said since I was still menstruating and not having hot flashes, it meant I couldn't be menopausal."

Marta tried a variety of herbal approaches and various supplements, including soy isoflavones, without any success and finally decided she needed to find someone who would look into possible hormone connections and check her hormone levels, since nothing else had worked and she seemed to be getting worse.

She said, *"I feel like I have no life right now. I get to live for about 4-5 days a month. The rest of the time I'm either in a social coma or feeling like I can't get out of bed."*

When I checked her hormones, her Day 1 estradiol level was low at 31 pg/ml, her total testosterone was also low at 28 ng/dl with a very low free testosterone at 0.6 pg/ml. Her thyroid profile was also abnormal, with a TSH of 7.2 and significantly elevated thyroid antibodies. All the rest of her metabolic and endocrine studies were in the desired ranges. She was perimenopausal, and had an autoimmune thyroid disorder. With these results, I wasn't surprised that she had been having problems with energy, weight gain, less endurance, and loss of muscle strength.

I started her on a combination of hormone therapies to correct these imbalances and loss of critical hormones. I suggested a bioidentical form of 17-beta estradiol, using a skin patch delivery, since a non-oral estradiol meant lower levels of SHBG, which would increase her available free, active testosterone. I thought the patch would also deliver a more optimal estradiol level in the range of about 90 to 100 pg/ml, which she would need in order to feel better.

She found she needed to change the patch every five days instead of the usual seven days it was supposed to last, because she was so physically active with her biking and running five or six days a week that she metabolized the estradiol more rapidly, and the patch didn't last a full week.

Fact:

Regular menses don't necessarily mean your hormone levels are OK!

Since her testosterone was also so low, and she had a noticeable loss of energy and muscle strength as well as loss of sex drive, I suggested she add bioidentical micronized testosterone in an oral sustained release tablet.

Since we don't yet have a testosterone patch approved for women, I have found that the compounded sustained release tablets are the next best option to help keep her energy level up over the course of the day.

Fact:

Too much soy can decrease thyroid *and* ovarian hormones.

With a TSH over 7 and such high levels of thyroid antibodies, she had Hashimoto's autoimmune thyroiditis, which no one had recognized. Her high soy diet was adding to the thyroid dysfunction and the ovarian hormone decline. I recommended that she cut out the soy foods and isoflavone supplements. She clearly needed thyroid medication, and I started her on an FDA-approved brand of bioidentical levothyroxine, or T4. Later on, I added a low dose of compounded sustained release triiodothyronine, or T3, until her TSH has reached the desired range of 0.5 to about 1.5. Her symptoms improved dramatically.

Within the first three months, she was thrilled that her hair had stopped falling out and was beginning to grow again. She also said, *"I have more energy and motivation, my memory is better, and I sleep so much more soundly now. I don't feel depressed like I did, and I feel my old spark is coming back."*

As her thyroid improved, her menstrual cycles became more regular. She was now making adequate progesterone, so we elected to wait a while before adding this.

She had also begun to lose that waistline "thickening," and was gradually seeing the excess pounds come off now that her thyroid and ovarian hormones were back into optimal ranges. She said her trainer had noticed that her muscle strength was now better, and she was responding more normally to her weight-training regimen. He asked her what she had been doing differently and she smiled and said, *"He was amazed when I told him what my new hormone regimen was and that I was taking testosterone. We both could tell that my muscles were getting stronger again with the exercises, like they always used to."*

She didn't have any adverse side effects on this dose of testosterone, and her cholesterol profile has continued to be in a healthy range. When I saw her recently, she said, *"I just feel better. I am back to the weight I always used to be, I have such good feelings of well-being and energy again. I just didn't realize how much I had lost until I got it back! I have been riding my bike more, and I really feel happy now."*

Another patient of mine, in her 70s, found that testosterone made such a difference in her energy and strength that she and her husband won their age group in a mountain hiking contest in Bavaria last year. I love helping my patients get their zest back by restoring hormone balance to complement all the hard work they are doing in taking care of themselves and trying to stay healthy and fit as they grow older.

Important!

Optimal estradiol is needed for testosterone to have its *desired* effects in women.

Testosterone and Brain Effects

I explained earlier how testosterone activates "sexual circuits" in the brain. It turns out, however, that testosterone is also a natural "antidepressant" hormone, along with estradiol.

Testosterone has significant "activating" effects on the brain, mainly by elevating brain levels of norepinephrine. These are the *same* type of brain activation patterns seen with the tricyclic antidepressants like desipramine, imipramine, or amitriptyline.

New research has shown that for testosterone to work properly in women, **an optimal level of estradiol must be present**. The brain testosterone receptor seems to be *created* by the presence of estradiol. Without enough estradiol to "prime the pump," even the testosterone produced by our own bodies cannot attach properly in brain centers. So, your level of estradiol becomes important here as well, since it also plays a critical role in how well your body's testosterone can work.

The bottom line is that our psychological sense of well-being is also enhanced by testosterone, in a synergistic way with the mood-elevating effects of estradiol. Both hormones contribute to positive moods when the amounts are present at optimal levels.

Studies going back to the 1930s have shown this mood-enhancing effect of testosterone supplementation in women, and the beneficial effects on mood were again confirmed in a 2003 randomized, double-blind placebo controlled crossover study using a transdermal testosterone cream.

Wisdom:

Too much tesosterone can be as bad as too little!

An Australian research study assessed the effectiveness of testosterone on mood and sexual function in otherwise healthy premenopausal women who presented with low libido and had documented low levels of testosterone. They found that treatment with transdermal testosterone cream improved the women's scores on the Sabbatsberg Sexual Self-Rating Scale, as well as scores on the Beck Depression Inventory, the Psychological Well-Being Index. There were NO adverse effects of testosterone reported in this study.

In studies from several different countries, testosterone significantly increased performance on cognitive tasks, in both women and men. Loss of testosterone in brain pathways as we get older is another factor in the onset of late life dementia.

How else do these brain effects make a difference for you if you have been feeling slowed, tired, or struggling with low sex drive? Think about all the times you have been to a physician for help with these problems and had the doctor tell you that you were depressed and then recommend an SSRI or tricyclic antidepressant to improve your energy and mood.

A hidden problem with these medicines is that all of them can increase your appetite for sweets and carbohydrate foods, and lead to more fatigue and weight gain. Did anyone check your testosterone and estradiol levels before suggesting an antidepressant?

Sadly, although psychiatrists in this country usually do check thyroid hormones, they have not been taught to check testosterone and estradiol levels when evaluating depressed patients so the *ovarian* hormone connection with depression and anxiety is missed. Women then end up having the undesirable side effects of antidepressants that blunt sex drive, *as well as still having the low hormone levels that were the major problem all along.*

It seems that in our current focus on antidepressant medications, we have overlooked the "antidepressant" effects of our natural hormones testosterone and estradiol that Mother Nature gave us eons ago! Not to mention, all their other crucial effects, as we have seen.

For women, testosterone effects on mood seem to have an optimal range at which the beneficial effects occur.

In my clinical work with women, I have found this optimal range to be of about 50-60 ng/dl for total testosterone, with a free testosterone of about 4-6 pg/ml. I find that levels lower than this are fairly consistently correlated with fatigue and depressed mood.

When testosterone levels are much higher than about 70 ng/dl in women, whether from over-production in the body or from taking too high a dose of hormone supplements, my women patients have typically described feeling more agitated, anxious, irritable, edgy, tense, angry, and don't sleep as well. They report difficulty falling asleep, increased dreaming and violent or aggressive nightmares.

At doses used by body builders abusing androgens for massive muscle building, *both* men and women develop toxic behavioral effects such volatile/explosive moods, aggressiveness, and assaultiveness. *Balance* is key.

Testosterone Effects on Sleep

Sleep becomes more fragmented and disrupted as we get older. Hormone changes play an enormous role in this, particularly the loss of estradiol. Sleep loss in turn

Vital News!

Mother Nature gave us "natural" antidepressants in our hormones!

disrupts the normal cortisol patterns and increases insulin release. These changes in turn affect your energy level and contribute to more weight gain at midlife.

The change in androgen-estrogen balance, and the usual higher level of free testosterone, that occurs when estradiol declines, together tend to make restless sleep even worse, since testosterone is a significantly stimulating hormone on brain pathways. If testosterone is given to women at bedtime, it can lead to fragmented sleep, violent or aggressive, disturbing dreams. Then you wake up feeling like you have been in a battle all night long.

Wisdom:

Testosterone normally peaks in the morning, and is lower later in the day.

Patients tell me that other physicians suggested testosterone be taken at night to help improve muscle repair. This theory isn't completely accurate. The activating brain effects of testosterone will disrupt Stage IV deep sleep, especially in women. This is the sleep stage for muscle growth and repair, and for release of Growth Hormone, which also affects muscle formation. If you don't get good stage IV sleep, you won't have much muscle repairing and building going on, no matter how much testosterone you have.

It is best for women, and men, to take testosterone in the morning to give you the desired boost to your energy over the course of the day, yet allow you to sleep more restfully at night. You will still get the beneficial effects on muscle repair and building if you take testosterone in the morning, and sleep better at night!

Testosterone and Hair, Skin and Eyes

"My eyes are getting so dry they burn." "I can't wear my contacts any more because my eyes are so dry, and I don't know what's causing this." I hear these comments often from women I see for hormone problems.

Many women haven't really considered that dry eyes can be caused by hormone problems. This symptom is extremely common in menopausal women, or in women who have had a hysterectomy leaving the ovaries. Both estradiol and testosterone have roles in keeping our eyes moist. Testosterone helps the mebothian glands in the eye make their lubricating secretions. If testosterone is too low, these secretions are reduced and the eyes are dry. Eye doctors often suggest a surgical approach using a "plug" to block the tear duct and help retain more moisture on the surface of the eye. To my way of thinking, however, it doesn't make much sense to plug the duct if no one has even checked hormone levels or tried restoring the hormone balance so the eye lubrication process works normally.

Androgens have marked effects on our hair growth, and are one of the primary regulators of how fast our hair grows, where and how thick it is. Paradoxically, androgens have different effects on hair follicles depending on whether they are in the body: they can stimulate growth of thick coarse dark hairs on the face, chin, back, arms, pubic area, or inner thighs; they can inhibit scalp hair follicles; they can have no effect at all on eyelashes.

Wisdom:

Hair growth
is affected
many
different
ways
by our
hormones.

It is one of those endocrine mysteries how one hormone can have so many different effects on hair. One reason may be that the hair follicle is one of a very few tissues in our body that can regenerate, and it often produces a new hair with different features. That appears to be one way that androgens affect hair quality in different areas of the body in different ways. It may also explain why sometimes you get a black, coarse hair on your chin, and then after plucking it, it may come back white and thinner.

Hair growth patterns in women can be profoundly affected by a variety of hormonal imbalances, both excess levels and hormone deficiencies. *Low* levels of androgens and estradiol, as well as thyroid and adrenal disorders, can cause loss of body hair, particularly eyebrows, underarms, legs, and pubic area. *High* androgen levels cause excess facial and body hair that is typically coarse and dark, especially if estradiol is also too low.

On the other hand, loss of scalp hair, called alopecia, can be caused by a several very different hormone imbalances, as the following list illustrates:

- ❧ Excess testosterone, DHEA, other androgens
- ❧ Androgen deficiency syndromes
- ❧ Loss of estradiol
- ❧ Excess progesterone relative to estradiol
- ❧ Excess thyroid hormones
- ❧ Thyroid deficiency syndromes
- ❧ Cortisol excess (Cushing's Syndrome)
- ❧ Cortisol deficiency (Addison's Syndrome, also called Adrenal Insufficiency)

Fact:

Too much money is spent on electrolysis to remove excess body hair, without getting a blood test first—it could be your hormones!

More Hormone Effects on Hair

To understand the many ways in which hair growth can be affected by androgens let's look at a few examples. If a woman's body is producing excessively high levels of DHEA, DHEA-S, and testosterone, she will often notice scalp hair *loss* at the same time she is having coarse, dark hairs on her face, chin, upper lip, around the breast nipple area, abdomen, inner thigh, arms and back.

Sadly, many women with androgen excess spends hundreds of dollars on electrolysis to remove excess body hair and never have had a single blood test of hormone levels to see if that's a cause of the problem.

If estradiol levels are too low at the same time androgens are too high, it accentuates these abnormal hair loss and growth patterns. Androgen effects on hair growth tend to be gradual, although if a woman is given too much supplemental testosterone, she may see rapid growth of excess facial hair. I will describe treatments for excess body hair later in the book.

Androgen deficiency syndromes, such as loss of testosterone with removal of the ovaries, leads to thinning and loss of both scalp and body hair. Women notice pubic and underarm hair disappearing, and notice that they don't have to shave their legs as often.

If estradiol is low, or thyroid hormones are too low or too high, the hair loss will be even greater. The loss tends to be gradual unless there is an abrupt loss of androgens, such as having the ovaries removed and having no testosterone replacement therapy. I find that if we get all these hormones back in optimal ranges, women start seeing hair on the scalp stop falling out, and body hair patterns become normal again. I remember when I was in my late thirties and having the early symptoms of low estradiol and falling testosterone, my hair started getting thinner, drier and more brittle. After being on good levels of both estradiol and testosterone for many years, my hairdresser has commented on how fast my hair grows and how thick it is now.

If you suddenly find yourself losing a lot of scalp hair, or having excess face and body hair, it is really critical to have your hormone levels—all of them—checked, and then consider treatment options I describe in upcoming chapters.

Testosterone and Estradiol Effects on Vulvar, Vaginal, and Urinary Problems

Women can experience many vaginal and urinary symptoms when estradiol and testosterone levels are too low.

Some of these problems include incontinence, urethritis, recurrent urinary tract infections, trigonitis, urethritis, urethral stenosis, interstitial cystitis, vaginal dryness, dyspareunia, vulvodynia, vestibulitis, recurrent vaginitis, often followed by a distressing odor and discharge.

Before I explain the effects of testosterone on vaginal and vulvar tissues, however, it's important to understand that the major effects are accomplished by estradiol with testosterone playing a complementary role rather than a primary one.

To keep healthy functioning of the vagina and urinary system it is important to have good estradiol balance before using vaginal testosterone cream or ointment.

Hormone Decline and Infections: In our premenopausal years, the healthy vagina has a slightly acid pH of about

Wisdom:

Both E2 and testosterone help keep vaginal tissues healthy!

4.5, and this acidic pH helps keep unwanted bacteria, such as those from the intestinal tract, as well as yeast from growing in the vagina and causing infections.

Once estradiol declines, especially if progesterone is still rising to its normal peak in the second half of the menstrual cycle, the pH of the vagina begins to be less acid and more alkaline.

Wisdom:

Changes in pH can cause more problems with infections.

When estradiol is too low, vaginal pH increases from the premenopausal level of about 4 to between 6 and 7. This change to an alkaline pH is a more favorable environment for unwanted bacteria and yeast to grow. The "good" bacteria, *lactobacilli*, aren't able to thrive and keep down the growth of yeast and undesirable bacteria like *E. coli* and others.

This is one reason you may experience more frequent urinary and vaginal infections as you get older or go through a period of hormone change. Optimal estradiol effect on the vaginal tissue keeps the pH acidic and reduces the growth of unhealthy bacteria. If estradiol blood levels are below the 50 to 60 pg/ml range, it is quite likely that this is a major cause of the urinary problems.

Undiagnosed diabetes is another very common cause of frequent urinary and vaginal infections in women, especially if you have gained a lot of weight.

Even before your fasting glucose is elevated to the level of diabetes, early stages of glucose intolerance can cause women to have more frequent vaginal yeast infections, itching vulva or vagina, burning on urination, increased urinary frequency, and even leaking of urine.

In patients I see for consultations, I find that low estradiol and testosterone levels and glucose intolerance or early diabetes are the most frequent *unrecognized* causes of persistent urinary problems

If you have a family history of diabetes, or have noticed an increase in craving for sweets, or have gained a lot of weight, you should talk with your doctor about more detailed tests for diabetes.

I have a chapter on this type of testing in my book, *Women, Weight and Hormones* (M. Evans, 2001). If you seem to be having recurrent vaginal or urinary infections, make sure you see your doctor for a urinalysis and urine culture before you start on antibiotics.

Don't just take antibiotics or Diflucan or over-the-counter yeast medicines thinking you know what you have. Repeated use of antibiotics and the anti-fungal medicines creates resistant bacteria and yeast organisms that lead to chronic infections.

I think it is also important to have your hormone levels checked. Many people still don't realize the degree to which loss of estradiol, and possibly testosterone, both play a role in causing these urinary and vaginal problems.

Work with your doctor to determine the possible hormone causes and correct the imbalances, perhaps first with a vaginal estradiol cream or vaginal ring. Then later consider adding a low dose testosterone cream if the estradiol alone doesn't fully take care of the problem.

For reasons we don't fully understand, the oral and transdermal estradiol used for the rest of the body, called *systemic therapy*, don't seem to give optimal effects on vaginal and bladder tissues. As a result, women with vaginal and bladder problems will typically need a topical estradiol tablet, cream or vaginal ring to improve the health of these tissues.

Hormone Decline and Vulvar/Vestibular Pain

Both testosterone and estradiol play a role in maintaining healthy levels of collagen that strengthens the vaginal and vulva tissue to prevent the thinning and tearing that occurs with loss of these hormones. Estradiol and testosterone play roles to improve vaginal blood flow and also maintain healthy levels of secretions from lubricant-producing glands in the vagina, and estradiol also helps to increase the moisture of cells in the vaginal

Wisdom:

Estradiol helps keeps a healthy vaginal pH.

and vulvar tissue. When the hormones levels are too low, you have more vaginal dryness, as well as more difficulty becoming lubricated during sexual arousal. This is another reason you have more itching and burning and sex becomes painful when the estradiol and testosterone are too low.

Both hormones also play a role in regulating pain pathways and nerve sensitivity, so if the estradiol and testosterone levels are too low, this causes you to be more sensitive to painful stimuli (i.e. the pain threshold is lower).

Wisdom:

Both E2 and testosterone play a role in vaginal lubrication and nerve sensitivity

At the same time, you will notice a deadening of sensitivity of the clitoris to sexual stimulation. Some women describe it by saying "I feel like I am numb, and don't feel stimulation of the clitoris like I used to."

In addition, decline in estradiol changes stomach pH to cause less absorption of calcium, zinc, and magnesium from dietary and supplement sources. Both of these minerals are needed as cofactors in the body's production of pain-regulating chemical messengers, so pain can intensify when there are low levels of calcium, zinc and magnesium.

Lichen sclerosus and *lichen planus* are two vulvar conditions that cause vulvodynia-type pain, severe itching and discomfort. These problems are more common in older women, but can also occur in younger women with low levels of estradiol and testosterone.

In my patients suffering from these problems, I have consistently seen improvement by using a topical low dose estradiol cream made without any preservatives, and sometimes I add a low dose (0.01% or less) of testosterone cream as well to help the tissues heal and repair.

Some authors have suggested higher dose testosterone (1 or 2%) creams alone, without estrogen. Because testosterone is so well absorbed from the vulva tissue, these doses are often too high and cause unwanted side effects of excess androgens like clitoral enlargement, voice deepening, acne, and mood changes.

Along this line, Joura and colleagues did a study of ten postmenopausal women with lichen sclerosus in which they used topical testosterone propionate 0.04 mg on a daily basis for four weeks. They found that even at this dose, *all* of the women had elevated serum levels of total testosterone and the level exceeded the upper normal range in *eight* out of the ten women.

The vulvodynia pain improved in nine of the ten women, but four women developed significant adverse physical signs of excess androgens. This is one reason I feel it is important to use estradiol cream with the testosterone, and to keep the testosterone dose low and make sure that testosterone blood levels don't go too high.

Caution:

Be sure that a testosterone cream dose is not too high.

Hormone Decline and Urinary Incontinence

It is a widespread misconception that urinary leakage, or *incontinence*, is an inevitable part of normal aging. It is not.

Incontinence isn't something you have to put up with as just a part of getting older. There are many approaches to helping this problem. I will talk about a few hormone aspects here, and then you can also read more in my book, *Screaming to Be Heard,* Revised Edition (M. Evans, 2001).

Continence is the ability to control urine flow, and hold urine in the bladder when you feel an urge to urinate. Once we are toilet-trained as children, most of us control urination urges unconsciously as we go about our daily activities.

Incontinence is the accidental loss of urine, or difficulty controlling the urine flow. Americans spend more than *10 billion dollars* annually on products to either hide the problem of incontinence, or to help them cope with it, without looking for ways to treat or eliminate the cause. The problem is even more widespread when you consider the prevalence in younger persons due to pelvic surgery such as hysterectomy.

The good news is that with modern approaches to treatment, better than 50 percent of incontinence patients can be cured, another 35 percent markedly improved, and the remaining 15 percent made more comfortable. Please do NOT sit home and suffer in silence if you have this problem.

When estradiol and testosterone decline, the bladder smooth muscle gradually loses its tone and strength. If the muscles of the bladder and sphincter aren't as strong, there is a decrease in the urethral closure pressure, which allows for more "leakage" problems.

Good News!

Incontinence can be treated. Don't suffer in silence!

Nerve endings also contain estrogen receptors. With normal estrogen levels, the sensory threshold is raised. When estrogen levels decrease, the sensory threshold is lowered, and the nerve endings become more sensitive leading to increased responsiveness to irritant stimuli that in turn contributes to an increased urge to void.

There is emerging research to suggest that testosterone with optimal estradiol is also needed to help maintain optimal muscle tone and strength of the connective tissue in the urinary system, and to also help maintain healthy vaginal tissue and clitoral sensitivity.

Let's now consider the types of incontinence and some hormone effects that may be important for you to discuss with your physician.

Stress incontinence is one you hear often, and patients are frequently confused about what it means. "Stress incontinence" does NOT refer to emotional factors causing loss of urine. It means the loss of bladder control due to the physical stress of increased pressure in the abdomen from such activities as laughing, coughing, sneezing, sexual orgasm, jogging, or straining during a bowel movement.

Stress incontinence is not caused by bladder spasms; it results from weakness or loss of tone in the bladder muscles, which is primarily due to mechanical factors, such as damage to the bladder muscles in childbirth.

It can also be caused by low estradiol and decreased testosterone that in turn cause weakness of the ligaments and muscles that help maintain bladder control.

Approximately 35 to 40 percent of younger women in their child-bearing years experience post-partum stress incontinence for as long as 6 to 12 weeks after childbirth due to trauma to the bladder muscles **and** the sudden drop in hormone levels after delivery. Stress incontinence is usually not associated with urinary frequency and urgency.

Urge (urgency) Incontinence is the sudden urge to urinate and not being able to hold your urine long enough to reach the bathroom. It usually results from bladder spasms.

Many cases of urge incontinence don't have a clear-cut physical cause, but it may also be caused by serious medical conditions such as herniated intervertebral disks, bladder infections, or by gynecological problems such as fibroids exerting pressure on the bladder or loss of optimal estradiol effect on urinary and reproductive tissues.

Urge incontinence is also aggravated by habits that cause increased urine formation, such as excessive fluid intake, alcohol, use of diuretics ("water pills"), beverages with caffeine, and/or tobacco use. It is important to see a physician for a thorough evaluation, because bladder cancer is also a cause of urge incontinence that has to be ruled out before proper treatment is started.

It is not a good idea to keep taking antibiotics for urinary tract infections (UTI), a common cause of urge incontinence, without having a careful medical evaluation to find causes that may need different treatment approaches.

Wisdom:

Estradiol and testosterone help maintain bladder muscle strength... and control of urinary flow.

Summary

As you can see, testosterone has effects on many body systems and functions, from your brain to your bones and muscles and more. It's a critically important hormone, and important to have checked as part of your overall health checkups.

But keep in mind for women, the balance of testosterone with estradiol is crucial to have all these systems working optimally, and to avoid the negative changes that come with too much testosterone. You can have low total testosterone and still have a relative androgen excess if free testosterone is too high, DHEA and DHEA-S are too high, and/or estradiol is too low.

It's the balance of all these that helps you feel your best. Don't start taking testosterone until you have your estradiol level checked to make sure it is also in the optimal ranges. I describe in later chapters ways to help you get checked and identify options to help you achieve a balance of these hormones.

"I feel so good! My recall is so much better now, I am really happy about that. The testosterone you added last time has really given me more get up and go. It also helped my energy, concentration, and focus. The vaginal dryness is better, too… not to mention my sex drive. This is great!"

— 48-year-old patient

Chapter 5
Dispelling the Myths and Misunderstandings

Myths abound. Misunderstandings permeate media stories. Testosterone has gotten a bad rap from the older high-dose preparations that were used for women, and from the abuse of androgens by elite athletes trying to "bulk up" their muscle mass and increase strength for competitions. "Estrogen" seems to always equate only with "Premarin."

Now we hear that "estrogen" causes cancer and heart disease and strokes. But did you ever wonder why young women with high estrogen don't die like flies of all these?

"Estrogen makes you fat, progesterone makes you lose fat." But did you notice that during your menstrual cycle you tend to eat more, feel more bloated and fat during the second half of the cycle, when progesterone is dominant?

We keep hearing that estrogen is bad, progesterone is good. Or that progesterone is a "wonder hormone" that cures all your problems. Or that testosterone makes you grow a beard, and makes your voice deep. We get urged to take DHEA, the "anti-aging" hormone.

But did you ever wonder how you "stop aging" and still manage to be alive?

No wonder women are confused. Every women's health book says something different. News headlines and articles only get part of the story—and usually focus on the most alarming part because scary headlines sell newspapers. No one seems to care whether they give you all the crucial information—we live in an age of sound bites, not in-depth reporting. Good news comes out later, and gets ignored.

FACT:
Premarin isn't the only estrogen. It isn't even "real" as far as what your body makes... it's the *horse's* mix of estrogens.

There seems to be little awareness that Premarin horse estrogens are markedly different from what our bodies make. Yet studies using only Premarin get generalized to all estrogens, and all ways to give it, even though we have studies going back 30 years showing how many differences there are among types of estrogen.

We also have studies showing that some risks, like blood clots, can be much lower when using the estradiol patch instead of a Premarin pill.

Wisdom:
Before you accept a diagnosis of "it's all in your head," have your hormone levels checked. *All* of them!

News reports of the December 2, 2004 FDA Advisory Committee meeting to consider the testosterone patch for women showed a number of such misunderstandings about hormone types and ways to deliver them when members of the committee based their delay in approval on findings from the Women's Health Initiative using Premarin and Provera.

Maybe you feel a little skeptical about what I have written so far. Maybe you are saying to yourself, "But, is testosterone really safe? Is it helpful? Do women really need testosterone? What about estrogen, do I really need it? Won't I gain weight from taking estrogen, or testosterone? What's the difference with all the types of hormones I hear about? How do I know what is right for me? How do I make sense of all this?"

I want to answer your questions with some key points to clarify these common myths and misunderstandings about hormones. I base my information on the extensive worldwide research over the last 50 years. I have read thousands of medical articles on these subjects, and I have attended national and international conferences where leading researchers in the world have presented their work. I can't cite all of these studies in the limited space of the Resource section; I have, however, listed key review articles and journals you may want to read.

I also refer you to my first book *Screaming to Be Heard* (revised edition ©2001), in which I provide more in-depth background information on these issues. Keep in mind that all of these ovarian hormones have key functions throughout the brain and body, not just reproduction. So to help you stay active, healthy, energetic, and feel sexy, you need to consider the balance.

Let's Set the Record Straight

Myth #1: *Testosterone and estrogen make you fat.*
**Fact: Taking hormones does not cause weight gain.
Loss of our premenopausal hormonal *balance* does.**

Whether it is too little estradiol, too little thyroid, too little testosterone, or too much insulin, too much cortisol, or an excess of androgens, it is the imbalance that leads to gaining fat around the middle of your body. The most important issue is balance. The right hormones, in the right balance for you, actually help you lose excess body fat more readily.

Myth #1:

Testosterone and estrogen make you fat.

Wrong!

The changing hormone balance during the climacteric or mid-life years takes many forms, but two are particularly important as they affect testosterone: (1) lower estradiol, higher estrone and (2) lower estradiol relative to the amount of testosterone present. These changes cause the testosterone effects to be "unmasked," so that you experience more of the male-like androgen effects on distribution of body fat, muscle mass, facial hair, voice, sex drive, and energy level.

Decrease in the estradiol at mid-life leads to a decreases in sex hormone binding globulin (SHBG). Since this carrier protein "binds" the sex hormones, having less of it means more androgens are now in the "free" or biologically active portion in the bloodstream.

At midlife, even if you have less testosterone and DHEA present than you did earlier, more of it is now active (free) form at the same time you have less of the feminizing estradiol effects…so you watch your body morph from a "pear" (gynecoid or female) pattern to the "apple" (android, or male) pattern of body fat, around the waist and "trunk" or upper abdomen/chest, growing more facial hair, and losing hair on the head.

It isn't just that you don't have the "willpower" to lose that middle spread; it is that your hormone ratios are now working against you.

The Post-menopausal Estrogen-Progestin Intervention Trial (PEPI) tested several hormone combinations compared to placebo in menopausal American women. The study lasted several years, so it could show long-term changes and effects on weight, metabolism, blood pressure, cholesterol, triglycerides, clotting factors and other variables. Even though women were given the types of hormones more likely to cause weight gain (Premarin and Provera), none of the hormone therapy groups showed a gain in weight.

The only group that gained weight was the placebo group taking no hormones. Recent studies from other countries, with various hormone combinations, show the same thing: postmenopausal women who don't take hormones consistently have more weight gain than women who do take hormones after menopause.

Myth #2:

Taking natural progesterone makes you lose weight. Testosterone and Estrogen make you gain weight.

Wrong!

Women who are not taking hormones after menopause also have a higher percent body fat even if their weight stays the same because they lose muscle when testosterone declines. Compared to women who do take hormones after menopause, women who don't take hormones also have more body fat around the waist and upper body, the risky "apple" shaped middle body obesity that leads to higher danger of becoming diabetic and developing heart disease.

Sadly, most women still don't know this and mistakenly think it's taking hormones that makes them fat.

Myth #2: *Taking natural progesterone makes you lose weight. Testosterone and Estrogen make you gain weight.*

Fact: The reverse is true: progesterone is the fat-promoting hormone to help you store fat for pregnancy.

Progesterone has several metabolic effects that lead to weight gain and more body fat, but here are a few major ones:

- It stimulates appetite so you eat more,
- It makes you less sensitive to insulin (i.e. more insulin resistant) so that your body stores more fat instead of breaking down fat for fuel,

ə It slows down the intestinal tract which allows you to absorb more calories from food (and also makes you feel bloated and constipated).

ə It down-regulates the estrogen receptors and blocks the testosterone receptors, decreasing your energy level to exercise.

Think about your own experience during your menstrual cycle. When do you get the hungriest and have food cravings? *Isn't it usually the week or ten days before your period?* This is when progesterone is the dominant hormone and estradiol is lower. Estradiol is highest the first half of the cycle, before ovulation, and progesterone is at its lowest during this part of the menstrual cycle. This first half, or follicular phase, tends to be a time of the cycle when women have fewer food cravings, and more energy to exercise.

Pay attention to your own body instead of the sales pitches for progesterone. Your body gives you the answer as to which hormone makes you have those uncontrollable hunger pangs and chocolate cravings!

Myth #3: *Hormones cause cancer.*

Fact: Hormones don't cause cancer. If that were really true, young women with the highest hormone levels would have the highest cancer rates. *This is not the case.*

Highest cancer rates are found in post-menopausal women. In particular, overweight or obese postmenopausal women have the highest rates of breast, endometrial, colon, and pancreatic cancers. Estrogen and progesterone may facilitate the growth of an existing cancer, but there is no data that shows either hormone *causes* cancers.

New studies with testosterone indicate a trend toward lower rates of breast cancer in women who take testosterone with estrogen after menopause. These studies suggest that testosterone may actually decrease cellular growth in the breast that can be stimulated by both estrogen and progesterone. While we need more information on this issue with longer-term studies, the preliminary find-

Myth #3:

Hormones cause cancer.

Wrong!

ings are certainly encouraging that postmenopausal use of testosterone doesn't increase women's risk of breast cancer, and may in fact, help to lower risk.

A recent study found no increase in risk of breast cancer in women using birth control pills. And there is even better news about the protective effects of birth control pills on two cancers: they reduce your risk of ovarian cancer by more than 50% , and your risk of endometrial cancer by more than 75% if you have been taking them five years or longer. So it isn't correct to say that "taking hormones causes cancer." In fact, the right hormone balance, along with healthy body weight, helps to keep your risk lower.

Myth #4:

All types of testosterone are the same.

Wrong!

Myth #4: *All types of testosterone are the same.*

Fact: No they are not. Methyl testosterone, is one form contained in older products like Estratest and recommended by some compounding pharmacists and physicians. *It is a more potent synthetic form of testosterone that in higher doses has been linked to liver damage and the formation of liver tumors.*

The German Endocrine Society banned its use in the 1980s for both men and women, but it is still in use in the U.S. for menopausal women. Bioidentical testosterone, without the added methyl group, is what I have used personally and for my patients for many years. It is made from soy and yam molecular "building blocks" (called precursors) and is available as a U.S.P. pharmaceutical grade powder. This powder can be made into a variety of delivery forms: tablets, capsules, creams, gels, suppositories, injection, and pellets.

Testosterone patches, lotions and gels for women that contain the natural form of testosterone are in clinical trials and being considered for FDA approval. Several pharmaceutical companies have other forms of testosterone products in development.

The bioidentical form of testosterone, usually in tablets or a low dose cream, is the one I recommend for my patients because I feel it gives better results with fewer unwanted side effects than I have seen with methyl testosterone.

Myth #5: *All estrogens are the same.*

Fact: No they are not. The 3 estrogens made by your body have important chemical differences and actions in the body, including different effects on your metabolism. *This is even more true for the plant estrogenic compounds (phytoestrogens, as in soy and red clover), synthetic estrogens (as in birth control pills), and the mixed, horse-derived estrogens such as Premarin (or it's plant derived, mixed estrogen chemical look-alike, Cenestin).*

Even though doctors prescribe these products and some women do fine on them, each of these estrogens contain different molecular "keys" and don't quite fit the "locks" of the estrogen receptors in our body the same way that our own 17-beta estradiol does. Consequently, many women don't feel as well on these other forms of estrogen as they do when using the bioidentical 17-beta estradiol options that are available in many forms of FDA-approved products as well as individually compounded ones.

Myth #6: *All progestins are the same.*

Fact: No they are not. Progesterone is the hormone made by your ovary. *Progestins are man-made ("synthetic") molecules that are chemically different from your body's progesterone.*

Some progestins are derived from progesterone (e.g Provera or medroxyprogesterone acetate, MPA) and some are derived from testosterone and called "androgenic" progestins (e.g Micronor or norethindrone), and some are derived from an androgen-blocking diuretic called spironolactone (e.g. drospirenone). This important difference affects their properties and the way they act in your body. Because they are so different chemically, if you don't feel well on one, you may do quite well on another.

For example, Provera is more likely to cause increased appetite, weight gain, bloating, breast tenderness, loss of libido and depressed mood compared to the androgenic progestins, like Micronor or Aygestin, which have fewer of these effects. But in some women, the androgenic progestins may cause more acne or irritability. Other women feel their best on the pro-

Myth #5:

All estrogens are the same.

Wrong!

Myth #6:
All progestins are the same.

Wrong!

gestin drospirenone because it helps to block excess androgen effects and also helps eliminate bloating due to its mild diuretic activity.

Myth #7:

All birth control pills are the same.

Wrong!

Myth #7: *All birth control pills are the same.*

Fact: No they are not. Different pills contain different ratios of estrogen and progestin, as well as different chemical types of progestins.

The higher the progestin (P) relative to the estrogen (E), the more likely you are to have increased appetite, weight gain, low sex drive, fatigue, headaches, and negative moods (irritability, depression). The better the E:P ratio, the less likely you are to gain weight or have trouble with "blood sugar swings". If your libido seems to have disappeared on your current birth control pill, talk with your physician trying a brand with a more estrogen and less progestin such as Ovcon 35 or Orthocylen.

Myth #8: *"Hormones don't help libido, you just need to see a sex therapist."*

Myth #8:

"Hormones don't help libido.

Wrong!

Fact: Doctors have really missed the boat here. Low testosterone has a significant role in causing low libido.

Doctors should check this before assuming you only need a therapist. Once your hormones, testosterone and estradiol, are in balance, a sex therapist may be an appropriate person to help you with a number of sexual problems. But, without hormones where they need to be for optimal function talk therapy won't be able to achieve its best level of success. An integrated approach, taking into account the biological/endrocrine *and* psychological aspects, is important.

Myth #9: *"You are too young to need hormones."*

Fact: Not true. Women of any age can have hormone imbalances that cause low libido and other problems like acne, weight gain, depressed mood, and fatigue.

The youngest patient I saw was an 8-year-old girl who suddenly "ballooned up" in weight with no significant changes in her diet or activity. Her DHEA was seriously elevated (in fact, she was on the way to having PCOS when she got older), and she also had elevated thyroid antibodies even though her TSH was normal.

As you read earlier, both of these hormone problems can cause rapid weight gain and low energy. I see many teenagers and young women in their 20s who have gained 30-60 pounds in just a few months with the serious hormone imbalances of PCOS. Even though many of these young women have excess androgens, they typically don't have high libido because their hormone balance is so out of kilter.

Myth #10: *"You couldn't have hormone problems, your FSH is normal."*

Fact: A high FSH (greater than 20) is a late stage in the transition to menopause.

Your levels of estradiol have been declining for several years before the FSH goes up, and if we only check FSH, we miss these earlier changes in estradiol, and testosterone as well.

Myth #11: *"You can't be having hormone problems, you are still having periods."*

Fact: Women can have lower than optimal estradiol and thyroid hormones and still menstruate.

Loss of menstrual periods is a late stage in the transition from our reproductive years to menopause. Whether or not you still have periods doesn't tell you very much about your testosterone levels, so it doesn't help answer questions about causes of low libido if you just look at whether or not you still have periods.

What you will notice, and what doctors often ignore, is that your periods are changing as your estradiol declines or your thyroid isn't optimal. When your estradiol declines, your flow is lighter, darker, and shorter in duration than when your estradiol is optimal. Periods stop altogether when the hormone decline or thyroid disease becomes more severe.

But long before your periods stop, you can have low estradiol and low testosterone causing your sex drive to plummet.

Myth #9:

"You are too young to need hormones."

Wrong!

Myth #10:

"You couldn't have hormone problems, your FSH is normal."

Wrong!

Myth #11:

"You can't be having hormone problems, you are still having periods."

Wrong!

Myth #12:

"You can't be having hormone problems, your vagina shows good estrogen effects."

Wrong!

Myth #12: *"You can't be having hormone problems, your vagina shows good estrogen effects."*

Fact: Women can have normal estrogen effect for vaginal lubrication and not have optimal estradiol for our sexual arousal and metabolic pathways.

Estrogen sensitive pathways in the brain appear to require higher levels to maintain normal function than do the estrogen receptors in the vagina.

Myth #13: *"I am too old to start hormones."*

Fact: You are never too old to feel better and have improved "hormonal health."

Myth #13:

"I am too old to start hormones."

Wrong!

There are a number of benefits from estradiol and testosterone, in particular, that can help you maintain healthy body composition, regardless of age. Some major ones are gain in lean body mass (muscle and bone), improved metabolic rate, improved energy, improved response to exercise, better balance, better memory, improved sleep (which lowers cortisol, improves Growth Hormone, allows muscle repair at night, etc.), improved insulin sensitivity, and better sexual response.

Healthy eating, exercise, not smoking... and can also help improve overall hormonal balance.

Myth #14: *"There is no need to check hormone levels because they vary too much."*

Fact: Not true. There is no greater variance in the lab tests we use for ovarian hormones than for the other standard lab tests we use, such as cholesterol.

Myth #14:

"There is no need to check hormone levels because they vary too much."

Wrong!

Besides, telling women we don't need to check hormone levels because they vary has to rank as one of the dumbest statements I hear physicians make to women! That's like saying we shouldn't measure blood pressure because it varies all day, or we don't need to check glucose in a diabetic because it varies. How do you know where you need to be if you don't know where you are? A 1998 study found that as many as 45% of the women on estrogen actually had serum estradiol levels below the thresholds for protective effects on brain, bone and other target organs, even though they reported their symptoms were relieved. The authors concluded that monitoring symptoms alone is not enough; assessment of serum hormone levels is crucial to insure adequate estradiol levels to provide the desired benefits.

Behind the Headlines

The "myths" I have discussed above are statements that are factually incorrect, and I have presented the medically correct information. But there are a number of hormone "misunderstandings" that arise when news headlines present only part of the story. For these, I have given you additional background to help address concerns you may have.

Misunderstanding #1: *"Taking estrogen after menopause increases your risk of breast cancer."*
Clarifications: The studies showing this increased risk have been ones in which women were using Premarin and medroxyprogesterone acetate (MPA), the *horse*-derived mixture of estrogens with a potent synthetic progestin that are chemically very different from the human 17-beta estradiol and progesterone. There are many studies showing no increased risk in women taking estrogen alone after menopause.

The U.S. Women's Health Initiative using Prempro is the primary study that media articles commonly cite, which showed a slightly increased risk of breast cancer in women on combined estrogen-progestin estrogen. Later, when further analysis of the data was done, this difference between the placebo group and women taking Prempro did not reach statistical significance, although this update was not widely reported in the media.

The authors of the study calculated that an individual woman taking Prempro had a 0.1% increase in breast cancer risk per year. An older Swedish study using estradiol valerate, a synthetic estrogen more potent than our natural 17-beta estradiol, initially reported in 1989 an increase in risk of breast cancer, but again, the follow up updated analysis in 1992 did not show any increase in breast cancer risk as they had initially thought.

Another older study, The U.S. Nurses' Health study, showed modest increased breast cancer risk, but what most media reports left out is that the increase in breast cancer was only found in those estrogen (Premarin) users who also drank alcohol, not in all of the estrogen users. We know that daily alcohol use is a separate risk factor for breast cancer.

Premarin gives high blood levels of horse-derived (equine) estrogens that are more potent than the human estradiol in their attachments to the estrogen receptors. These horse estrogens are not easily metabolized by our body's enzyme systems and therefore, the longer you take them, the more potential there is for them to build up in the breast tissue.

These oral estrogens in Premarin are also more potent in stimulating the liver to make more SHBG, which then lowers your free testosterone and can lead to loss of libido and more fatigue.

For all these reasons, I don't feel Premarin is the best estrogen option for *human* females!

Misunderstanding #2: *"Testosterone can cause liver damage."*
Clarifications: This is based on use of the synthetic methyl testosterone in oral form, and at significantly higher doses than we use today for women.

These problems have not been seen with proper physiologic replacement with bioidentical testosterone that does not have the added methyl group, which appears to be the culprit causing liver damage. If you are concerned about possible adverse effects on the liver, using a nonoral form of testosterone (cream, gel, patch, injection, or suppository) reduces this possibility even more.

Misunderstanding #3: *"My libido is still low, I need more testosterone."*

Clarifications: Not necessarily. Just adding more testosterone may not produce any improvement in sexual desire, and may actually interfere with normal sleep, mood and pain regulation as well as cause more middle body weight gain.

There are some interesting findings from recent research on sexuality in women: (1) women need optimal levels of estradiol in order for the brain testosterone receptors to work properly in stimulating the sexual desire-arousal circuits, so it is important to optimize your estradiol before adding testosterone; (2) women, more so than men, are sexually aroused by the quality of the relationship to an even greater degree than being aroused as a result of their hormone levels. Male sexual response is more purely "biologic" than women's. Female sexual desire clearly has biological components related to levels of estradiol and testosterone, but for many women, the emotional-intimacy connections are an even greater part of becoming sexually aroused.

Misunderstanding #4: *"I don't have any symptoms, so I don't need hormones."*

Clarification: Both symptoms and health risks should be included in your decision-making.

Don't focus on just whether you have symptoms. The crucial issue is whether you are missing silent, subtle changes that may be significantly affecting your health, such as low energy, loss of muscle, low libido, abdominal fat gain, bone loss, brain effects (memory loss, sleep disruption), and many others.

You need to assess these other factors with the testing that I describe. Then consider: Do I need hormones or not? If yes, which hormones will help improve which symptoms and which health risks? Which symptoms or health risks may be made worse by the wrong type of hormones? Which type and route of taking hormones is best suited to my needs and preferences?

Misunderstanding #5: *"I went through menopause smoothly, I don't have hot flashes anymore, so I don't need hormones."*

Clarifications: This is similar to the comments I made in #4.

You may not have hot flashes any longer, but are you losing energy? Has your interest in sex disappeared? Are you gaining weight? Do you feel sluggish and foggy-brained? Then you may have some of the effects of low estradiol and low testosterone.

Take a look at the results of your lab tests, and see if there are any imbalances that could be helped with proper hormone balance. All these other body-brain changes may be a reason to consider hormone therapy, regardless of whether you have hot flashes.

Misunderstanding #6: *"I'm 65, so my doctor told me to stop my hormones."*

Clarifications: For the same reasons I described in #3 and #4, reaching a particular age is no reason to stop hormones if you have been taking them and feeling well.

Remember, in addition to bone loss, our loss of muscle and memory, along with gain in body fat, gets worse the older we get unless we address the hormone imbalances that perpetuate these problems. As a result, older women may be in greater need of the benefits of hormone therapy than younger women.

Besides, who said you are too old to feel well...and sexy, and have zest and vitality to do all the things you want to do now?

Misunderstanding #7: *"Estrogen and the birth control pill cause blood clots."*

Clarifications: The estrogen data on this issue was based on oral estrogen, primarily Premarin, and use of birth control pills in women who smoked cigarettes.

Newer data on the patch (transdermal) form of estradiol, our bio-identical premenopausal estrogen, shows that estradiol actually decreases the risk of thrombophlebitis ("blood clots") through a number of mechanisms that I described in detail in *Screaming to Be Heard*.

Cigarette smoking is a separate risk for blood clots and strokes. Re-analysis of the old data, separating women into smokers and non-smokers, showed that non-smokers taking BCP did not show this higher risk of blood clots and strokes.

The older studies were also based on the older, very high dose (>100 mcg of ethinyl estradiol and 1-2 mg of progestin) formulations used in the 1960s. None of those high-dose pills are even available today. Today's BCP formulas are a fraction of the hormone content used when the pills first came out. **About 1990, BCP were FDA-approved for use in non-smoking women over age forty because the potential benefits far outweighed risks.**

Misunderstanding #8: *"Everybody I know takes Prem-Pro. Why should I try something different?*

Clarifications: Every woman's needs are different. Your body is different, your genes are different, your metabolism is different, your health issues are different, as is your lifestyle.

If hormone therapy is truly individualized, you would not expect to take exactly the same amount and type as your friend takes. It's crazy for so many doctors to continue this "cookbook," "one-prescription-fits-all" approach to women's hormone needs that has been the standard approach in the United States for decades. It's equally nonsensical for you to buy into faulty logic when your health is at stake. Besides, why would you want to take something Mother Nature gave the horse, instead of the exact hormone molecule Mother Nature gave you?

Misunderstanding #9: *"HRT doesn't prevent heart disease."*

Clarifications: This headline is based on "The Heart, Estrogen-Progestin Replacement Study (HERS) Study," and doesn't take into account serious shortcomings of the study itself.

These are (1) the women already had heart disease with

blockage of the coronary arteries when the hormones were started; and (2) the hormone product being used was PremPro, a combined product of horse-derived estrogens and a potent synthetic progestin (MPA). None of the women were given estrogen alone, or a bioidentical form of estrogen, to compare a natural estradiol with estradiol plus synthetic progestin.

To everyone's surprise, including the researchers, women taking the combined hormones had 50% more heart attacks than women taking placebo, and 3% more clotting problems in the first year of the study. This is what the news articles focus on, leading to the "misunderstanding" above.

Critical Points Overlooked in the News

To put this information in better perspective, let's look at key points:

- (1) During the last two years of the study, women on the combined HRT had 40% fewer heart attacks, more consistent with many studies that show hormone therapy reduces heart disease risk over time;

- (2) HERS participants taking combined HRT had an 11% reduction in LDL ("bad") cholesterol and a 10% increase in HDL ("good") cholesterol. These were positive changes, though not as good as the improvements in cholesterol measures seen when estrogen (particularly 17-beta estradiol) is used alone, or is used with natural progesterone instead of the synthetic progestin MPA.

- (3) It takes on average, about 1.5 to 2 years before a reduction in cholesterol will show a decrease in heart disease risk. The women in the HERS trial were not in the study long enough to see the full benefit of hormone therapy.

But there are other serious problems with the HERS design. In the 1970s and early 1980s, British researchers Drs. Campbell and Whitehead showed that the horse-derived estrogens had the potential to have much worse effects on heart disease risk measures than our own natural 17-beta estradiol. Even though the negative effects of Premarin and Provera (combined to make PremPro) have been known over twenty-five years, the HERS designers still chose to use the horse-derived estrogen and the synthetic progestin.

Progestins like MPA reduce the beneficial effects of estrogen on a number of heart disease risk factors, such as the good cholesterol levels, blood vessel wall "elasticity," fibrinogen levels and others. The PEPI Studies, published in 1995, showed that bioidentical progesterone did not have the same negative effects on cardiovascular measures as MPA. But the HERS designers still chose to use only the synthetic progestin in the study. To those of us who have long advocated use of more natural forms of hormones for women, it was actually encouraging news to see our concerns demonstrated so clearly in the HERS Study results.

Take Home Messages

- If you already have heart disease, or its risk factors, I suggest you avoid using a continuous combined horse-derived estrogen and synthetic progestin product like PremPro.
- If you are already on PremPro and have problems with weight gain, high blood pressure, high triglycerides, glucose intolerance or diabetes, insulin resistance, high cholesterol or a history of heart problems, I suggest you talk with your physician about changing to the bioidentical human forms of estradiol and progesterone.
- Transdermal 17-beta estradiol, alone or with natural progesterone (for women with a uterus), has better benefits on these metabolic pathways and fewer adverse effects on SHBG to lower your free, active form of testosterone.

A Final "Misunderstanding": Dealing with Your Insurance Plan

Insurance companies in the United States express concern about the growing health care costs today. One example often cited is that obesity increases risk of diabetes, high cholesterol, high blood pressure, heart disease, breast and endometrial cancers. They have extensive databases showing that obesity is a far greater problem among women than among men, and that this gender discrepancy commonly begins following a woman's first pregnancy. Yet, the hormone factors that play a role in women's weight gain are rarely addressed. The balance of estradiol and testosterone is a critical factor, and doesn't get checked.

We get letters from "managed" care insurance plans on almost a daily basis in both of our medical offices asking us to change our prescriptions to one of their "preferred formulary" prescriptions. Preferred formulary medications are typically older, cheaper, often generic, versions of medications that may be similar, but not necessarily identical to, the product that you and your doctor have decided you should take. Your insurance carrier is doing this to save money. They pressure doctors into changing your prescription medication to one that costs them less, regardless of whether it is as effective or may cause more side effects.

Case Study: Patti's Story

Let's look at an example from my practice: A 39-year-old woman requested my help to identify triggers of her low libido, hormonally-triggered migraines, and weight gain. Her gynecologist had started her on Demulen birth control pills in hopes this would help her PMS, but her migraine headaches began soon after, her libido plummeted, and her weight ballooned upward. Her doctor tried another brand of pills without success. Then her prescription plan said she had to change to a "preferred formulary brand" (Nordette or LoOvral) if she wanted reimbursement, so she tried them. All of the BCP she tried made her headaches and weight gain worse.

The headaches became so severe she required care in the emergency room to break the migraine cycle. By the time I saw her, she was pretty desperate for relief. The BCP had also depressed her mood, and sex drive. Her physician recommended she see a counselor.

Needless to say, she was understandably fed up with the whole idea of birth control pills, and said, "I guess I'll have to try and put up with the PMS, because if I don't find a way to lose this weight and get my headaches under control so I don't miss work, I will lose my job. If I don't get my libido back, I'll probably lose my husband too!"

I explained how the estrogen and progestin ratios in these brands had worked against her. These brands are all higher in either dose or potency of the progestin. High progestin pills aggravate headaches, and cause low libido as well as trigger more weight gain than low progestin pills that have a better balance of estrogen (ones like Yasmin, Ovcon 35, Orthocyclen, or Modicon). Her own health insurance plan had made her problems worse by insisting she use these high progestin pills.

The health plan's required formulary products also resulted in increased cost for her medical care:

(1) she now needed more prescription medications for her headaches,

(2) she now needed medicine to control high blood pressure caused by the high progestin pills,

(3) she had numerous ER visits to treat acute, severe headaches, and

(4) she now needed medicine to treat the blood sugar problems caused by the weight gain.

So, did the insurance company really save money? Of course not. And this list doesn't include the cost to the woman herself as she had to buy new clothes as her weight escalated out of control, or the pain and anguish she suffered as she watched her body shape change, her self-image plummet and her marriage suffer.

It is true that all these brands had similar safety profiles and similar effectiveness at preventing pregnancy, but they have profound differences in side effects and effects on appetite, metabolism, weight gain and headaches.

Pharmacists often say to us "They are the same, it is only 5 (or 10) micrograms difference in the estrogen," or "It is only a half milligram difference in the progestin." Such small differences in progestin can be profound for many women and lead to major differences in how the pills affect you.

Summary: Be in Charge—Speak UP!

Speak UP!
You may
be the only
person to
advocate for
you and your
health.

You deserve better, so speak up when your insurance plan is trying to get you to change to a "preferred formulary" product. You can insist on being given more information about what the differences may be and how this could affect other problems you may have. If you try a formulary product and it causes more problems for you, and your plan doesn't allow you to use a product "off formulary", then file an appeal (using the process outlined by your health plan) and push to be allowed to use safer and more effective products that work for you.

Hormone imbalance at mid-life has important implications for your health and well-being. I've taken you through the facts behind the myths and misunderstandings. It's now time for you to make the decision that you feel is right for you. If you are fed up with feeling dead-tired all the time, tired of having no sex drive, frustrated with feeling so blah every day, then check your baseline hormone levels as I outline and go step-by-step through the options I describe to help you make sound decisions about getting your hormones back in balance.

Tap into *your* hormone power.

Chapter 6

Old Approaches to Testosterone Therapy

Various testosterone therapy options for women have been around for over forty years, but it has only been in the last decade or so that we have seen more widespread use of testosterone for women. You have probably heard many of the fears about bad side effects of testosterone as I have mentioned in earlier chapters.

How did these fears get started? What were some of the problems with the older forms of testosterone? What were some of these older products and what were some of the problems? How do they differ from "natural" testosterone options that I recommend for my patients? Let's explore these questions and shed some light on the scary tales you may have heard about testosterone.

FACT: Women make more testosterone than estrogen for *all* of our reproductive lives

What's the Difference between Synthetic and "Natural," or Bioidentical Testosterone?

The word "synthetic" has come to be used as if it meant "artificial" or "foreign chemical" or "something different from what the body makes," but this is not a correct use of the term.

"*Synthetic*" simply means "produced by synthesis. Synthesis means putting together building blocks to make something, and synthesis can occur in a biological organism (human, plant, animal) or it can occur in a laboratory.

Hormones that are exact copies of what our body makes can be *synthesized*, or produced, in the laboratory much like a locksmith copies your master key to make a duplicate key for your home or car. Scientists have figured out how to make exact copies of many of our hormones: human insulin, human growth hormone, human thyroid hormones, human adrenal hormones, as well as bioidentical forms of human ovarian hormones. All of these have been made commercially by pharmaceutical companies into products that are used throughout the world to help overcome various kinds of hormone problems. These are examples of *synthetic* (i.e. made in the laboratory) medications being used because they are the exact duplicates of ones found in human bodies.

Because the human body does not have the enzymes to change these plant precursors into the ovarian hormones, the chemical precursor molecules are extracted from the plants, purified, and then synthesized in the laboratory into molecules *identical to those made in the human body.*

We call such molecules *bioidentical* when they are exact copies of the human form of the hormone. Even though such bioidentical hormones are made in a laboratory by "synthesis," rather than in a natural biological organism, that does not mean they are artificial or any less like the ones our own body makes. Molecules that are the same as those made by the body, even if synthesized in a laboratory, are generally better tolerated, more effective, and have fewer side effects than hormones that are different from our own body forms.

Conversely, the estrogens found in Premarin are "natural" because they are made by a biological organism (horse), and the estrogen-type compounds in soy are natural because they are also made by a biological organism (plant). Neither of these estrogens are bioidentical, exact copies of the human 17-beta estradiol.

Scientists have also invented compounds that are unique and are chemically different from those made by the human body. These compounds are also made by "synthesis" in the laboratory, and can also be called "synthetic."

Wisdom:

Bioidentical hormones made in a lab by "synthesis" are still "natural" because they are exact copies of our own body hormones

In the case of compounds that are *not* like body molecules, "synthetic" does mean "different from the body hormones," or "artificial."

Some examples of these are medroxyprogesterone acetate (MPA) or Provera, ethinyl estradiol (used in birth control pills worldwide), methyl testosterone, and others. These are "synthetic" hormone medications that are truly "artificial" in the sense that they are chemically different from the molecules the body makes, even though they may have some similar effects to the ones our bodies make.

So I think it ends up being confusing to use the term synthetic when talking about hormones. I feel it is more important to differentiate whether you are describing compounds that are bioidentical to those in the body, or compounds that are chemically different. And then decide which type may be needed for a given health reason. There is a place for each type of compound in trying to help women achieve various health goals.

For example, contraception needs the potency of the "synthetic" chemically different estrogens and progestins that can suppress ovulation; bioidentical estradiol and progesterone don't provide reliable contraception, and may in fact, be used to enhance fertility.

Women with endometriosis often need the potency of "synthetic" or novel progestins to help suppress pain from endometriosis. Menopausal women, on the other hand, often feel better and have fewer side effects when using the bioidentical hormones.

Some authors and some physicians claim that only compounding pharmacists can make "bioidentical" hormones. Others claim that big drug companies don't make bioidentical hormones because they can't patent the natural molecule and make money on them. **These claims are blatantly false.**

Scientists at large pharmaceutical companies were the ones who originally identified and purified the hormones estradiol, progesterone, and testosterone in

Wisdom:

Premarin may be "natural" for a horse, but *not* for a human!

the 1930s. It was the large pharmaceutical companies that identified ways to make these bioidentical ovarian hormones from yam and soy plant molecules, and purify them to make raw powder of what we now call U.S.P. pharmacological grade estradiol, progesterone, and testosterone. This raw powder then becomes the source for everyone else, *including compounding pharmacists*, to make their various pills, potions and patches. So it's important for you to realize that the raw ingredients all come from the same place for the major pharmaceutical companies and the small pharmacies to use in making products.

All of the hormones made by the ovaries are extremely large molecules that are inactivated or destroyed by digestion when taken orally. This is one reason that in the early days, companies doing hormone research developed chemically different molecules like medroxyprogesterone acetate and methyl testosterone. These chemically different hormones could survive the digestive system and be active when taken as oral tablets. Once the process of *micronization* was developed in the 1970s, and these large steroid hormone molecules could be made into particles small enough (*micronized*) to survive digestion and be absorbed into the bloodstream, commercial pharmaceutical companies could begin to make tablets, patches, gels and creams of bioidentical hormone products.

Methyl **testosterone** is an example of a form of testosterone created in the laboratory and not found in the human body. Methyl testosterone was developed by scientists trying to find a way to make testosterone able to be used in an oral tablet. In the past, we did not have a way to give bioidentical testosterone orally because it would be broken down and lost in the digestive process before getting into the bloodstream. The methyl group on testosterone makes it possible to be absorbed orally without being completely lost in the digestive tract first. Once absorbed, it can then produce testosterone effects at the receptors throughout the brain and body.

Fact:

The testosterone patch that is currently in clinical trials contains bioidentical testosterone, not methyl testosterone.

But, it is also this methyl group that increases the potential for liver toxicity, including forms of liver cancer. Liver toxicity was seen primarily in men using methyl testosterone because the doses for men were higher than those used for women. The German Endocrine Society recommended over twenty years ago that methyl testosterone not be used for men or women because of the potential risk with long term daily use.

Once the bioidentical hormones have been synthesized, they can then be made into standardized forms so that you and your doctor know the amount of hormone you are getting. Using standardized, pharmaceutical grade products, I feel, allows better "fine-tuning" of hormone therapy than trying to get enough active hormone from plant/herbal sources, since you really are not able to determine how much you are taking, and whether the amount is right for you. And you don't know what other compounds in the plant may *not* be good for you either.

Today, we have a wide variety of bioidentical hormones that are all FDA-approved. Examples include Estrace tablets, generic estradiol tablets, estradiol vaginal cream, Vagifem vaginal tablets, Femring and Estring vaginal estradiol rings, Estrogel and Estrasorb estradiol skin lotions, estradiol patches (Climara, Vivelle DOT, and generic ones), Prometrium progesterone tablets, Crinone and Prochieve vaginal progesterone, injectable progesterone, estradiol and testosterone, etc.

Pharmacists can also formulate bioidentical testosterone into in a wide variety of other forms: skin cream, skin gel, oral sustained release tablets, sublingual tablets (to dissolve under the tongue), and vaginal suppositories.

The way that testosterone is given will determine (a) the amount absorbed, (b) the metabolism to different forms, (c) the development of desirable effects, as well as (d) the presence of adverse side effects. I generally don't recommend the rapidly absorbed forms of testosterone such as gels and sublingual tablets or troches,

Wisdom:

Bioidentical hormones do not *have* to be made by compounding pharmacists; they can also be obtained by prescription from your local major drugstore pharmacy.

since these are more likely to make you feel like you have been hit by a Mack truck when the blood levels rise so fast. A rapid rise in testosterone to high levels typically causes marked irritability, edginess, muscle tension, aggressive, angry feelings.

I have listed in the Appendix some experienced, reputable pharmacists who will work with you and your physician to determine the proper amount of natural testosterone for you, provide educational resources and telephone question/answer services to assist patients and physicians in determining the most appropriate options.

Smarts:

Unwanted testosterone effects are decreased by using either oral sustained-release testosterone, or a low dose slowly-absorbed cream form.

My Response to the Myths About "Male Hormones" for Women

Most of the women I see have already heard comments like those I made at the beginning of this chapter: testosterone causes a mustache, a beard, deep voice, liver damage, and "oversexed women." A key factor most women don't know, because it isn't addressed in books and magazine articles, and doctors have not been taught this: all of the above problems are related to the *dose* and *type* of testosterone used, not just testosterone itself. In the U.S. until very recently, we have only had synthetic *methyl* testosterone or other androgen compounds that are not made in the human body.

These chemically different androgens are much more potent than the natural hormones made by the ovary and adrenal gland.

Until more recently, doctors did not realize that women needed *much* lower doses of testosterone than had previously been thought, because amounts were figured based on doses used for men. In the United States, we have not even had commercial, FDA-approved tablets available in doses *low* enough for women.

As an example, in the past, Premarin with methyl testosterone contained either 5 or 10 mg of methyl testosterone. This is far more than we use today, even when using the less potent form of micronized bioidentical testosterone, much less the potent methyl testosterone.

On average, I am using doses of 0.5 mg to about 3 mg a day of oral bioidentical testosterone. Obviously, this is quite a difference from what was usually contained in the old preparations. These lower doses are based on the physiologically natural range of testosterone production in women.

When using a more appropriate *woman's* dose, my patients tell me they feel more energy, have a return of their normal sex drive, and do not have the unwanted side effects described above. In addition, I monitor cholesterol blood levels and have not had any patients who have had a negative effect on their cholesterol levels if we keep the dose in the usual range for women, and check to see that blood levels are not getting too high.

Fact:

Women need much lower doses of testosterone than previously thought.

Currently, there is a natural testosterone patch in a dose designed for women that has been developed with the same technology that has made estrogen and progestin patches available. The published data so far from the clinical trials shows very promising results for both safety and effectiveness to improve libido in women. At the FDA Advisory Committee meeting December 2, 2004 to consider whether to move toward approval of the testosterone patch, committee members asked for additional long term safety data, which means it will be likely another year or longer before we have this option available for women.

The FDA-approved **male** testosterone patches should not be used for women because they contain much too high a dose for women to use, even if you cut them into little pieces. Androgel, the FDA-approved **male testosterone gel** product, also contains far too much testosterone to be safely used for women.

Future directions for androgen research in the United States are focusing on the role of testosterone in

Alzheimer's disease, in improving cognitive function in older people without dementia, in treating bone loss for men and women, in lipid disorders and breast cancer.

With greater recognition of the important role testosterone plays in many aspects of our health as men and women get older, and the benefits and safety documented in the initial studies of the transdermal testosterone patch for women, it would be helpful if we could move more rapidly toward getting FDA approval for a woman's patch form of testosterone.

Problems and Pitfalls with Compounded Testosterone Products

Until we have an FDA-approved form of bioidentical testosterone such as the patch, we only have non-FDA approved options available from compounding pharmacies to use for women who need testosterone added to their hormone regimen. I have used such compounded products successfully since the mid 1980s, but I have also seen such products misused and women overdosed with excessive amounts of testosterone when doctors and pharmacists don't seem to know how to determine the proper dose.

So, here are some important cautions you need to know when using tablets and creams that are made up to individual prescriptions rather than being manufactured in set doses, regulated by the FDA.

Many popular books and authors have been recommending a "1%" testosterone cream (or gel) for women, and some even suggest "2%" creams or ointments are appropriate for women. These doses are way too high for women, and can lead to seriously elevated serum testosterone levels, as well as multiple adverse effects, such as hair loss, acne, muscle pain and spasm, insomnia, anxiety, agitation, weight gain with middle body fat deposits, high total cholesterol, low levels of good cholesterol.

Wisdom:

Men and women require *different* amounts of hormones.

Male testosterone patches and gels contain far too much tesosterone for women.

To put these doses in perspective, 2% testosterone ointment or cream contains 20 mg per gram. One gram is ¼ teaspoon. This means each day, a woman using ¼ tsp. of a 2% testosterone cream is getting **20 mg** of testosterone. This is a dose used for *male* testosterone replacement. The usual conversion is that non-oral forms of medicines should be about 1/10ᵗʰ an oral dose. So this means that if a woman is getting 20 mg of testosterone in a non-oral cream, it would roughly the same as taking 150-200 mg ORAL testosterone, clearly an excessive dose. Remember, I typically recommend 0.5 mg to 3 mg daily with oral testosterone, or 0.1 mg to 1.0 mg in non-oral form.

Caution!

1% and 2% creams of testosterone are too high for women!

Likewise, a 1% testosterone cream or gel contains 10 mg per gram, and one gram is ¼ tsp. So if you are using ¼ tsp. of this compounded 1% product, you would be getting 10 mg of non-oral testosterone a day, roughly the same as taking a 100-mg tablet form of testosterone, which again is a *male* dose. As I mentioned above, I usually use only 1-3 mg of oral micronized testosterone —quite a difference!

If you use a cream, using the same guidelines as the testosterone patch that is currently in clinical trials

How will you know if you're getting too much testosterone?

- Excessive or unwelcome sexual thoughts and drive
- Aggressive or violent dreams
- Irritability, difficulty sleeping
- Acne, oily skin, facial hair
- Loss/thinning of scalp hair as in male-pattern balding
- Muscle tightness, soreness or spasms
- Uncontrollable food cravings
- Upper body or waist area fat
- Increased blood pressure
- High cholesterol   © Elizabeth Lee Vliet, M.D. 2005

and contains 300 mcg (0.3 mg) of testosterone, the correct dose for a cream would be 0.1 to 0.5 mg of testosterone per gram of cream or gel, **not 10-20 mg per gram**. Then when women use 1/4 tsp. of testosterone cream, she would be getting 0.1 to 0.5 mg of testosterone a day, or about the equivalent of about 1-5 mg oral testosterone a day.

When I use the testosterone cream in these doses, I get blood levels that are in the physiologic replacement range, just as has been published for the testosterone patch studies.

When I have tested women's testosterone levels when they were using 1-2% testosterone creams from another physician, I have gotten total serum testosterone levels ranging from 150 to 600 ng/dl, clearly in the MALE range and completely inappropriate for women. No wonder the women I have evaluated who are using such high dose compounded testosterone products have so many problems.

Wisdom:

Compounded testosterone cream for women should be ~ 0.1 to 0.5 mg/gm, on average.

The following women show some of the difficulties that excess testosterone can cause, whether it occurred from the body making too much testosterone and DHEA, or whether they were taking a dose that was too high for a woman.

Toxic Testosterone Cream

I was shocked when I received the lab reports on Lydia, a pleasant 46-year-old woman. Her total testosterone was *586 ng/dl with a free testosterone of 109 pg/ml*. I thought at first I had misread a decimal point! A woman's total testosterone should be about 50-60 ng/dl, but 586? That's a healthy level for a man! Yet her estradiol was only about *half* what it should have been at the midpoint of the second half of her menstrual cycle.

I checked her chart to see what she had been taking. Her former physician had prescribed a compounded 2% testosterone cream to be used 2-3 times a week. This blood level was drawn *24 hours* after she had last applied the compounded cream, so in fact, her testosterone level had been much higher the first several hours after she put the cream on her thigh and vulva. I was dumbfounded. I had not seen a woman's testosterone level that high in all my years of medical practice.

What was even more interesting to me is that she still described having low libido and "disabling fatigue" daily, in spite of such excessively high testosterone levels. My experience tells me that a key reason her libido and energy level had not improved with even high dose testosterone is that she had not been given any supplemental estradiol to restore this hormone to its optimal level for a woman. **I have consistently found that women can have high testosterone levels—produced by their body or from taking large doses—and not get the usual benefits of testosterone if the estradiol is too low.**

Here are her words to describe how she felt:

Caution!

10-20 mg/gm testosterone creams can give blood levels in the MALE range!

> "I am very tired, with very little energy. I have a hard time thinking logically or clearly, concentrating and interacting with people. I can force myself to carry on a brief conversation but doing so increases my symptoms. At the worst, I feel lightheaded, almost dizzy, but if I close my eyes and try to relax, I don't fall asleep. I have hot flashes and nighttime sweats, I get very emotional and cry over little things. I have been having more problems lately with aching joints, my muscles hurting all over, and I don't sleep well. I never had problems like this until I hit this menopause thing. The gynecologist I see doesn't usually treat women with male hormones, so she just did what the pharmacist told her to do for the testosterone. I'm not feeling right, but I am not comfortable adjusting my dose without the supervision of a doctor who knows more about all this."

At her consult, her physical exam showed some changes that occur with excess testosterone. She had very thick, dense, coarse pubic hair in a diamond shape like a male pattern, not the typical finer pubic hair in a triangular shape characteristic of the female pattern. Her labia were darker in color, and the clitoris had enlarged slightly. Her good cholesterol had dropped to 39, much lower than typical for women of her age and health status, and she also had gained more fat around her waist, giving her a waist to hip ratio more like that seen in men. All of these changes were typical of androgen excess.

Wisdom

Low E2 + excess T = many problems!

She elected to start on the Climara patch, and I asked her to stop the high dose testosterone cream until her level came down. At her follow up appointment two months later, she said, *"I am thrilled at how much better my digestion is since I started the estradiol. My energy is better, my mind is clearer, I feel more alert, and my memory is better. The hot flashes and night sweats are gone, and I am sleeping better."*

Her testosterone had now dropped to 21 ng/dl, so she wanted to go back on testosterone in a more appropriate dose. I suggested she try a sustained release oral 1 mg tablet to give her better stability in her energy level over the day, and not last so long that it would interfere with sleep. She liked this approach, and has done well on the combination of the estradiol patch, oral low dose bioidentical testosterone, and cyclic low dose progestin every two months. The androgenic changes in her body and lab results have all improved.

Androgen Overload

Lynda was a 35-year-old mother of triplets who had been seeing a fatigue and fibromyalgia specialist and was on a complicated array of hormones, psychotropic medicines, supplements and herbs when I first saw her. She had a severe viral illness at age 15 and was diagnosed with fibromyalgia at age 22. She had trouble getting pregnant and then had 3 miscarriages in a year. No one had checked her hormone levels until she finally saw a fertility specialist. After many tries, she became pregnant and at age 30, delivered triplets. She decided to have a tubal ligation because she felt she couldn't endure another miscarriage or the emotional and financial strain of more infertility treatment.

Not long after her tubal ligation, she began having migraine headaches which she had never had before. She also experienced worsening muscle aches and severe fatigue. The specialist she consulted started her on a whole pharmacopeia of medications at the outset: thyroid, cortisone, estradiol patches, progesterone cream, testosterone cream, DHEA, Ambien for sleep, SOMA and Neurontin for muscle pain, Klonopin and Flexeril to help relax her sore muscles, Nystatin for yeast, Provigil to improve her energy, and a variety of digestive enzymes and other supplements. In addition, she had difficulty keeping the Climara patch on, so the fatigue specialist told her she could stop the estradiol patch and increase the progesterone.

The longer she continued the higher dose of progesterone, the more painful her ovulation became and the heavier her periods became. Finally, her Gyn recommended she have a hysterectomy. He was able to spare the left ovary, but said it had been full of blood and needed to be drained at the time she had her surgery. She was 34 years old. After her hysterectomy, her Gyn recommended she stop the testosterone and progesterone to see how her remaining ovary would function.

Not surprisingly, it didn't function very well, and her hormone levels plummeted. She decided to go back on the testosterone cream, which was now formulated to contain 2.5 mg of testosterone, 100 mg of progesterone, and 0.125 mg estradiol and estrone, with 1 mg estriol. She was using this cream twice a day, which meant she was getting double these amounts of each hormone. While the estradiol amount in the cream was quite low, both the progesterone and testosterone amounts were too high for non-oral delivery.

To put it in perspective, the FDA-approved bioidentical progesterone cream for vaginal use delivers 40 mg every *other* day or an average of 20 mg once a day, not the 200 mg a day she was getting in the compounded cream.

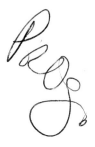

Caution!

Don't start too many new medicines all at once... you're likely to have more side effects!

The testosterone patch that is currently in clinical trials delivers 300 mcg (0.3 mg) testosterone daily, NOT the 5 mg a day Lynda was getting in this compounded cream. I wasn't surprised she was having so many mood and physical problems.

At her consult with me she said,

> *"My doctor didn't do any hormone tests, so I don't know where I am. But the last several weeks I've experienced extreme irritability, exhaustion, and a deep depression. My muscle pain is terrible, and the migraines are back and I can't function because they are so frequent and so severe. I can barely get through my days and take care of my children. I am really worried about all the medicines I am taking. Even with the sleeping pills, I don't sleep well and I wake up exhausted in the mornings. I am too young to feel this way, and I am frightened by how bad I feel."*

Caution:

High dose progesterone creams can cause severe fatigue and depression

I was quite concerned about all the medications she was taking, some of which—Klonopin and Flexeril—I felt were actually making her fatigue worse. The high dose of progesterone in this cream also contributed to her fatigue and depression, especially since she wasn't getting nearly enough estradiol to balance all the progesterone. With her uterus removed, there really was no medical reason for her to even be taking progesterone. The high dose of testosterone in her cream was causing more muscle spasm and tightness, as well as causing insomnia and irritability. The low dose of estradiol in the cream, as well as the rapid rise and fall with this cream delivery system, was a major culprit in her migraines being so much worse. Then there was also the problem that the more medicines someone is taking, the more there are side effects and drug interactions to deal with.

Her hormone levels confirmed my suspicions. Her total testosterone was far too high for a woman at 268 ng/dl, when it should be only 40-60 ng/dl. The blood level was drawn 2 hours after the cream was applied, and the level had only dropped to 148 ng/ml at 24 hours after she used the cream.

The constant high testosterone level contributed to her insomnia, irritability, and muscle spasms. Her estradiol was only 72 pg/ml, too low in general, but especially with a testosterone this high, which was another reason she wasn't sleeping well and felt so tired and depressed.

The hormone cream gave her a progesterone level in the ovulatory range at 6.5 ng/ml. This would also have been much higher in the first several hours after she applied the cream, which was why she felt so exhausted and depressed in the mornings after she put on the hormone cream.

Her DHEA was several times higher than desirable for a woman, and her thyroid was over suppressed with the dose of Armour thyroid she had been given. The combined excess DHEA and thyroid further added to her insomnia, irritability, palpitations, and muscle aches.

I told Lynda and her husband that it would take some time to gradually wean her off the excessive number of medications and find a balance of hormones and delivery methods that would help her regain some stability. Painstakingly over the next year, we worked together on finding a hormone regimen that worked for her and tapering her off the multiple medications. It took about 10 months, but she finally stabilized on the Vivelle DOT estradiol patch with a vaginal estradiol ring to help prevent vaginal dryness, and a daily dose of 2 mg oral sustained release bioidentical testosterone tablets. She did not need DHEA or thyroid.

Over several months, I was able to help her taper off all the other medications for pain and sleep now that her hormone balance was optimal and her levels back in the desirable ranges.

She consulted a new migraine specialist who was able to treat her migraines with just a low dose of amitriptyline 25 mg at bedtime for a daily preventive medication, and an occasional Fioricet to treat pain when a headache

Caution:

High dose testosterone creams can cause irritability, muscle pain and spasms, and insomnia occurred. Now that her hormones were more stable, she didn't have nearly as many migraines as she had been having when I first saw her.

It is a tribute to both Lynda and her husband that they persevered through a long ordeal to get her off the excessive medicines and find a hormone regimen that worked for her and restored healthy levels of both estradiol and testosterone. *Balance* is so critical when restoring women's hormones to optimal levels.

Hormone Havoc

"I felt like an alien has taken over my body."

Too Much Testosterone

When I first saw her, "Risa" was 17 and in anguish, feeling betrayed by a body that was felt like it was careening out of control—pounds going on so fast she couldn't fit in last month's new clothes, uncontrollable food cravings, pimples popping out like gangbusters, hair growing everywhere it wasn't wanted—face, neck, arms, inner thighs, back, wild mood swings that went from angry outbursts to tears in a flash.

She described feeling like an alien had taken over her body, and nothing was working. Her trainer couldn't understand why her diet and exercise regimen no longer kept her weight down, her family was at a loss to understand her mood changes and outbursts, and their daughter who used to sleep through a thunderstorm was now waking up multiple times a night and then feeling exhausted in the mornings. Her school work was deteriorating and her teachers had commented on the marked behavior changes. Her primary care doctor, thinking she was a depressed adolescent, recommended she see a psychiatrist. The psychiatrist tried multiple antidepressants, but nothing seemed to help, and she only felt more wired and anxious on the medications.

Her mother began to suspect a hormone problem after noticing that her daughter's periods had become so irregular, but her gynecologist just told her that her daughter needed to eat less and exercise more. Both mother and daughter were intensely frustrated by the time I saw her for her consult.

In addition to the physical changes in her body with the marked increase in body and facial hair, the acne scars, and the male pattern to her pubic hair, her hormone levels told the story of the "alien" that had overtaken her body. Her androgens were extremely high and her estradiol was as low as we typically see in menopausal women.

It's as if a male "alien" had taken over a female body and usurped the normal female endocrine control. Let's look at her numbers compared with a healthy female balance:

	Risa's values	Optimal female values
Total testosterone	81 ng/dl	40-60 ng/dl
Free testosterone	20 ng/dl	4-7 ng/dl
Free + weakly bound	37 ng/dl	10-15 ng/dl
Testosterone DHEA, unconjugated	1093 ng/dl	200-400 ng/dl
Estradiol, day 19	32 pg/ml	200-250 pg/ml
8 AM cortisol	25 µg/dl	10-18 µg/dl

Wisdom

Anti-depressants don't work very well when hormones are this much out of whack!

The rest of her baseline labs were in healthy ranges, including all of her thyroid tests. So it was clear that her ovaries were making too much testosterone and DHEA, and these excess androgens were causing her mood and physical changes.

Since her estradiol was so low and her androgens were so high, I recommended that she start a birth control pill that had a better level of ethinyl estradiol relative to progestin to help reduce the side effect of weight gain.

The combined estrogen and progestin in the pill would further help decrease the excess DHEA and testosterone by suppressing her ovarian hormone production. I also suggested she take spironolactone, an androgen-blocking medication used to help treat excess body hair in women. I suggested she continue to work with her trainer for her exercise and healthy diet.

A few months later, her androgen profile was now in the desirable range, with total testosterone now at 30

Wisdom:

The oral estrogen in the BCP would help to counteract the negative effects of the androgen excess by increasing liver production of SHBG and binding up the excess free testosterone.

ng/dl, free and weakly-bound (bioavailable) testosterone decreased to 11 ng/dl, free testosterone of 6 ng/dl, and DHEA now at 400 ng/dl. Since she was taking a birth control pill that provided ethinyl estradiol, which isn't measured by the usual lab tests, I did not recheck her estradiol because I knew she would be getting an adequate amount of estrogen in the birth control pill. Her 8 AM cortisol had now come down to a more desirable level of 15 µg/dl. All in all her numbers had improved greatly, even though the androgens were still higher than what we typically see in women taking oral BCP.

She was pleased when I saw her again at her follow up appointment—her acne had cleared up well, her excess facial and body hair had decreased markedly, her mood was more stable, she had lost 15 pounds and was having a much easier time staying with her diet and exercise routine. Her mother reported that she no longer had the wild mood swings like she did, and how that she was sleeping so much better, her school performance had also come back up to her usual A level of work. She was much happier now that she was feeling more like her old *female* self.

Commercial Testosterone-Estrogen Combinations:

Estratest®: esterified estrogens..........................1.25 mg (oral tablets)
                and methyl testosterone............2.5 mg
Estratest® HS: esterified estrogens..................0.625 mg (oral tablets)
                and methyl testosterone............1.25mg
Depo-Testadiol®: estradiol cypionate............2.0 mg (injectable)
with testosterone cypionate..........................50.0 mg

Discontinued by the manufacturer, approximately 1997:
Premarin® with methyl testosterone (MT).0.625 mg E, 5mg MT
....and 1.25 mg E, 10 mg MT

Problems with Combo Products

Premarin with methyl testosterone had far too much testosterone for most women, particularly when you consider the much lower dose of estrogen included in the tablet, and the fact that Premarin delivers such a small amount of the most active form of estrogen, 17-beta estradiol. Since these high doses of testosterone were commonly used in the past by the dominant estrogen manufacturer, I think this is one of the primary reasons that oral testosterone therapy got such a bad name and was associated with so many unwanted and potentially serious side effects.

I have *never* used even 5 mg of oral methyl testosterone, much less 10 mg of this more potent form of testosterone, in prescribing androgen therapy for women.

Doses this high of methyl testosterone for women may commonly cause development of facial hair, acne, voice changes, loss of scalp hair (male pattern baldness), elevated total and LDL cholesterol, decreased HDL ("good") cholesterol, elevated triglycerides and insulin, as well as more body fat deposited around the waist.

If your doctors are concerned about such side effects when you ask about testosterone therapy now, it is likely that they are remembering what happened with the older forms and higher doses of testosterone therapy. They may not realize that micronized testosterone, in the bioidentical ("natural") form the ovaries made, is only about 1/3 to 1/4 the potency of methyl testosterone, and we are using much lower doses today than what used to be contained in older products.

The brand Estratest has become much more popular and widely used in recent years, thanks to increased awareness by physicians and consumers of the importance of testosterone for women. Although this product can be fine for some women, I think there are problems with this product you need to keep in mind. Estratest contains esterified estrogens that, when you take it orally, are converted primarily to estrone. As you recall, estrone is the estrogen produced in body fat and in the ovaries and liver as a reservoir for the ovaries to make estradiol. Estratest delivers very little of the desirable 17-beta estradiol, and it also contains the more potent artificial form of methyl testosterone, not bioidentical testosterone.

Since Estratest doesn't deliver an adequate amount of 17-beta estradiol to properly balance the amount of testosterone it contains, many women tell me that when they started Estratest, they began to have problems with acne or oily skin, flare-ups of fibromyalgia pain, irritability, insomnia and feeling anxious or tense, not sleeping well, and hair loss.

Caution:

Combination drug may seem convenient, but *may* cause more problems because they are not *your* balance.

Such problems, in my experience, occur when there is an excess of testosterone relative to estradiol. I am not surprised to hear these negative comments from women who try Estratest and decide not to continue.

Estratest illustrates another common problem with any medication that comes in a fixed dose combination of different hormones or medications. There may not be enough of one thing and too much of the other for everyone to have the right blend. As a result of these problems, I rarely use the *fixed-dose* combination estrogen-testosterone. In my opinion, these fixed-dose products do not allow for individualized adjustments of hormone therapies tailored to each woman, which is the way I think it should be done for best results.

I find it works much better to adjust each hormone separately so that you get exactly the right amount of each hormone for your body needs. Taking each one separately also allows you to make changes in only one at the time, based on what you are experiencing with desirable or undesirable effects, or interactions with other medications (such as antibiotics, asthma meds, etc.) or effects of situational stresses on your hormone metabolism.

If, however, you want to have the convenience of a combination estrogen-testosterone tablet available at your local drugstore or you want a prescription that is more likely to be covered by your health insurance, sometimes women do fairly well by first starting a 17-beta estradiol prescription (patch, gel, or tablet) and then use Estratest HS just 2 to 3 times a week rather than every day. This approach minimizes the adverse side effects of the higher dose, more potent methyl testosterone and yet provides a more optimal and consistent level of 17-beta estradiol than is provided by Estratest. This approach seems to work well for some women.

Some women find they can use these combination products daily and experience the desired benefits without unwanted side effects. But if you have tried Estratest and it caused side effects, perhaps you now understand why this might have happened. You can try options that give you better levels of estradiol and bioidentical testosterone.

Wisdom:

Your "hormone recipe" will be slightly different from your friends. The key is finding what is best for you.

Cautions

- ❧ Make sure estradiol has been restored to optimal levels before adding testosterone

- ❧ You should not take testosterone if you are pregnant or nursing, or are trying to become pregnant

- ❧ You should avoid oral testosterone if you have a history of liver problems

- ❧ Testosterone doses should be kept in low range to give blood levels similar to those of the menstrual cycle.

- ❧ Avoid high dose testosterone creams and products designed for men.

Chapter 7
DHEA: Promises and Pitfalls

Dehydroepiandrosterone, or DHEA is widely promoted today as an "anti-aging" hormone. With all the publicity DHEA has had in recent years, manufacturers have scrambled to sell a wide variety of DHEA products, of varying quality and potency, to aging baby boomers looking for the magic fountain of youth.

FACT:

OTC DHEA products rarely deliver on their health claims.

You can find DHEA products all over the country, widely available on supermarket, drugstore and health food store shelves, over the Internet, and in health product catalogs, not to mention the multi-level marketing companies that also include it in their product line. DHEA is recommended by many alternative and "natural hormone" practitioners as the "Mother Hormone" precursor for the body to make estradiol and testosterone, even though there are major flaws in their theories, as we shall see when we explore this further in the sections that follow.

There are no controlled clinical trials showing that DHEA meets these promises, yet it is still widely promoted for many conditions, from low libido to memory loss and is suggested by some authors as the way to treat fibromyalgia or chronic fatigue. Remember, these are *marketing pitches* to *sell* over-the-counter supplements, and they are all outside the regulatory purview of the FDA that restricts what manufacturers of *prescription* medicines can say in their ads. You can't believe all you hear with OTC supplements.

Caveat emptor! **Let the buyer beware.**

A key problem with all the books and sales pitches that hype DHEA is that the authors, for the most part, have failed to take into account two critical issues:

(1) The claims of DHEA benefits are based on experiments in rodents with a fundamentally different DHEA physiology:

(a) Rodents produce miniscule amounts of DHEA, so when DHEA is given to animals in studies, it is something being *added* they don't normally have.

(b) Doses used in the animal studies are often much greater (i.e. *pharmacologic*) than what would be appropriate *physiologic* "replacement" for humans, so we don't know whether we are seeing results that occur only with high doses or not.

(c) The animal model is also flawed, since animals don't go through the same decline in adrenal androgens (*adrenopause*) that humans do.

As a result, most researchers studying DHEA in humans question whether the data from rodents is applicable to humans. Studies in humans so far do not show the same benefits seen in rodents.

(2) The claims of DHEA slowing down the ravages of aging assume similar effects in human men and women, ignoring critical differences between men and women's biology in the way DHEA is processed by the body, and fundamental differences in the impact of varying estrogen-androgen balance for each gender.

Almost all of the studies showing that DHEA may have promise as an "anti-aging hormone" have been done either in *men* or in rodents.

Another significant problem is that over-the-counter DHEA is a food-grade product, not the pharmaceutical grade used in prescription products used in reputable research studies. The FDA does not regulate over-the-counter DHEA products as they do for prescription hormones, so there is no quality control or standardization to insure that you are getting what the label says

Caution:

OTC DHEA products are NOT the same quality as pharmaceutical grade used in research studies the product contains. Not only is it difficult for you to know exactly what you are getting when you buy it, it is also a big problem that most of the doses being used are much higher than *women* need for daily use. More isn't always better, especially when dealing with androgens and women's bodies.

Reputable studies by respected researchers show that studies giving DHEA to men and women with age-related, natural (i.e. *physiological*) decline in DHEA show no specific, consistent benefit compared to placebo.

Even in women and men with various symptoms, Buvat pointed out in a 2003 review of many studies of DHEA that there has not been any consistent benefit of DHEA found in *any* placebo-controlled trials, except one involving women over age 70 that I will describe below.

There are a few specific situations, such as Addison's Disease, in which DHEA shows potential benefit for women, and I will describe those studies later in the chapter.

But DHEA has potential problems for women, such as a lowering of our "good" HDL cholesterol, which could potentially increase risk for heart disease. Women given doses of DHEA higher than about 30 mg a day also commonly experience virilizing (i.e. masculinizing) effects of oily skin, acne, facial hair and voice deepening.

There is also a darker side to the DHEA story for women: some studies suggest a potential increased risk of breast cancer in women using supraphysiologic doses of DHEA.

Remember women's basic biology: you have to have *functioning* ovaries for the "Mother Hormone" to be made into estradiol and testosterone. Most of our current research points to these as the critical hormones for the benefits we seek, such as improved memory, better sex drive and sexual arousal, improved sleep and energy, improved lean body mass, improved well-being. It is less likely that it is DHEA that provides these

Wisdom:

You have to have *functioning* ovaries for the DHEA to be made into normal amounts of estradiol and testosterone.

effects. If you have had a tubal ligation, hysterectomy, or have become menopausal, then your ovaries aren't functioning optimally to carry out all the conversions needed for DHEA to become the important "end" hormones, estradiol or testosterone. Taking DHEA in these situations can lead to androgen excess, with all the typical unwanted effects I have described earlier. It may ultimately be safer and simpler to directly restore the lost estradiol and testosterone since we know much more about their effects in women.

Caution:

DHEA use
has many
pitfalls for
women.

Don't be
duped
with hyped
claims.

With so many headlines, magazines articles, and books touting the benefits of DHEA on everything from brainpower to better sex, it is amazing that there is so little good science to back up the claims. This situation is very different from the extensive body of science showing the many beneficial effects of estradiol for women, and the extensive data on the possible risks and benefits that we need to be aware of when considering long-term use of various types of estrogens, testosterone and progestins.

DHEA use is definitely encumbered by a great deal of controversy. What dose of DHEA is safe? What are the long-term risks of taking it? Are there any benefits unique to DHEA itself, or are the observed positive findings due to it's conversion to estradiol and testosterone? These are critical unanswered questions. This is a far different situation from what we have today with so much good information available about doses, routes of delivery, risks and benefits for estradiol, testosterone, progesterone and progestins.

So, before you jump on the bandwagon and buy your "superhormone" at your local grocery or health food store, remember this is a potent steroid with profound effects throughout the brain and body. I will explain problems that can occur with taking daily DHEA, as well as potential benefits of DHEA that have been found for certain types of disorders. Read further, get properly tested, and make sure you have done your homework before you swallow all the claims...or the pill!

What is DHEA and Where Is It Made?

Scientists first identified DHEA-S in urine in the 1934, but it wasn't able to be isolated from the bloodstream until 1954. The biological function of DHEA and DHEA-S remained largely unknown until the 1990s. In fact, because DHEA had so many puzzling scientific aspects, and so many unanswered questions, it was the topic of a 1997 international conference of world experts on DHEA, sponsored by the International Health Foundation. I have summarized in this chapter some key findings from that conference as well as from more recent research.

DHEA occurs in two forms in the body:

(1) *unconjugated* DHEA (or DHEA non-sulfate), primarily made in the ovary and testes and also made by the adrenal glands, and

(2) *conjugated* DHEA or *DHEA-sulfate* (DHEA-S) that is the major steroid secreted by the adrenals, occurring in larger amounts than cortisol. DHEA and its partner, DHEA-S, are made from the basic building block of cholesterol, in a series of steps that include intermediate molecules called pregnenolone (sulfate) and 17-hydroxypregnenolone.

These initial steps take place primarily in the adrenal glands, and then the final steps synthesize DHEA in the ovary and testes from intermediate compounds.

DHEA is also one of a number of steroids made in the brain, called *neurosteroids*, synthesized in nerve tissue directly from cholesterol. These neurosteroids can be found in the brain *even after removal of the ovaries, testes or adrenal glands*, which helps confirm that the brain pathway is independent of the endocrine glands in the body. In fact, some of the newer studies have shown that levels of DHEA and DHEA-S in the central nervous system are 5-10 times higher than levels found in the bloodstream, and may directly affect certain brain functions. Studies in rat brains suggest that DHEA

Wisdom:

DHEA occurs in two forms in the bloodstream.

Both are important to measure.

increases nerve cell excitability by actions at the GABA receptor, but there is much more that needs to be clarified about its role in the human central nervous system. This is an exciting area of research today to uncover the role neurosteroids play in mood, memory, attention, sleep, pain and other functions, particularly with regard to male-female differences in response.

FACT:

DHEA varies over the day, while DHEA-S remains more steady.

Both DHEA and DHEA-S circulate in the bloodstream, but DHEA-S is strongly bound to the carrier protein *albumin*, while DHEA is only very weakly attached to albumin. These binding differences mean that women especially may see unwanted androgenic effects from higher levels of DHEA since there is more in the free, active form. The concentration of DHEA-S in the bloodstream is about ten to twenty times the amount of cortisol, also made by the adrenal glands.

On average, a young adult man or woman makes about 25-30 mg of DHEA-S per day. DHEA (non-sulfate) is typically about 500-1000 times *lower* in the bloodstream than the concentration of DHEA-S. Studies have found that the average young adult makes about 2-7 mg of DHEA per day.

DHEA-S levels in the bloodstream are more constant over the 24-hour day than is DHEA. DHEA shows pulse type variations in secretion similar to the pattern of cortisol, with higher levels in the AM and lowest levels in the late afternoon. That's why some physicians say that measuring only DHEA-S is more reliable, but I find that it is important in women to know levels of both forms, especially if they are having symptoms of androgen excess.

Until very recently, both DHEA and DHEA-S were considered only *precursors* or *prohormones* that did not have specific hormonal effects themselves, but exerted their effects only by being converted to the end hormones estradiol and testosterone. To be classed as a true *hormone*, a compound must have an identified receptor site specific for that molecule and none had been found for DHEA or DHEA-S.

But new research, published by Liu and Dillon in 2002, described a newly identified DHEA receptor on the membrane of endothelial cells lining the aorta in cows. Williams and colleagues also published a study in 2002 that suggests there may be a specific DHEA receptor in human smooth muscle cells lining the walls of blood vessels. DHEA didn't bind well to the estradiol and androgen receptors also found in vascular smooth muscle cells, but did show a strong attachment to this new type of receptor. As a result of these findings, our ideas and understandings of DHEA are changing rapidly.

DHEA Patterns Through Our Life Cycle

FACT:

Yes, DHEA declines as we age... but so do estradiol and testosterone.

DHEA starts being produced during our fetal life, then levels fall drastically after we are born. About age 7-9, during what we call *adrenarche,* the adrenal glands again start making more DHEA-S and DHEA in both boys and girls. DHEA levels peak in the late teens and early twenties in both males and females.

Levels then begin a progressive decline in men and women. But most studies show that after the age of about 50, DHEA-S levels are about 10-25% lower in women than men. By the time we reach about age 70, DHEA levels are only about 10% of what they were in our peak reproductive years. In premenopausal women, the adrenal gland produces about 90% of our DHEA-Sulfate, which is in a dynamic balance with DHEA. DHEA is produced by both the ovary and adrenal gland before menopause, and then after menopause almost all of the DHEA-S and DHEA are made by the adrenal gland in lesser amounts.

We know that a number of medical disorders *cause* low DHEA and DHEA-S. Examples include Addison's Disease (Adrenal Insufficiency, described later), hypopituitarism, therapy with corticosteroid medications, chronic illness, and severe or prolonged emotional or physical stress.

So we don't yet know for certain whether low DHEA levels seen in older people are *caused* by health problems like diabetes, autoimmune disorders, life stress, etc. or whether the decline we see in adrenal androgens (adrenopause), represents just an effect of getting older. There may also be the possibility that the *decline itself* causes the problems we thought were due to aging, such as loss of muscle strength, loss of optimal immune function, loss of cognitive "sharpness," loss of bone and many other effects. But since the studies are so confusing and conflicting in their results so far, no one knows for certain at this point which it is.

Wisdom:

Men and women require *different* amounts of DHEA.

We *are* different.

DHEA: Concerns and Cautions for Women

DHEA use has some special concerns and cautions for women that I want to briefly address here. I don't have space to go into all the pros and cons, or to describe in detail the research findings.

I will cover the highlights, and if you would like to read more about DHEA from well-respected DHEA researchers, I recommend articles by Dr. Peter R. Casson, MD and Professor A.R. Genazzani (Italy), which should be available on-line and in libraries.

Both researchers give a balanced and reliable view of what we know and what we don't yet know about the safety and effectiveness of DHEA for women. Dr. Casson has been researching DHEA in human females for many years, and has published a number of well done studies. Professor Genazzani is an expert on neurosteroids; his articles are a reliable resource for you to read if you want more in-depth information than I have been able to provide here.

In human studies, important differences for men and women are emerging. A 1988 study on five young men by Nestler and colleagues showed that these young men given high dose oral DHEA over a month had a decrease in body fat and a decrease in "bad" (LDL) cholesterol. That was a positive finding that has not been repeated in subsequent studies. The data on DHEA and cardiovascular effects *in women* continue to be conflicting.

Mortola and colleagues then conducted the same study in women: *no benefits* were seen. In fact, the women became "androgenized" with increased face and body hair, acne, decline in good (HDL) cholesterol and increase in bad (LDL) cholesterol, decreased sex hormone binding globulin, and *increased* insulin resistance.

Remember, insulin resistance helps make you fatter around the middle of your body and increases your risk of diabetes and heart disease—not a good thing cosmetically or from a health standpoint.

In addition to the possibility of weight gain with excess DHEA, there is a concern emerging from animal studies about possible adverse liver effects of long-term oral DHEA use, particularly at the high doses being promoted for women in the over-the-counter products.

Dr. Casson did a subsequent follow up study using a much lower dose of DHEA (50 mg) for women and found that even this dose (commonly seen in over-the-counter products) caused excessively high testosterone serum levels in women and androgenic side effects. He reported that this finding indicated the need for further dose reduction if DHEA was being given to women.

Earlier studies suggested a cardio-protective effect of DHEA. Again, this was in men and the positive effects were *not seen in women*. In fact, the decrease in "good" HDL cholesterol seen in women given DHEA suggests a negative effect on cardiovascular health.

Two groups of studies suggest that DHEA can have adverse cardiovascular effects in women: (1) those of postmenopausal women with high DHEA-S showing that they have a higher risk of heart disease than women of the same age who have lower levels; (2) young women with PCOS with high DHEA-S levels

Caution:

DHEA can have adverse heart effects in women... unlike what studies show for men.

also have a higher risk of heart attacks in their 30s and 40s, much younger than usually seen in women.

As I mentioned earlier, DHEA, like other precursor or "building-block" hormones, requires enzymes found in healthy ovaries for the DHEA to be changed into testosterone or estradiol by the body.

Caution!

Too much DHEA is dangerous.

Don't overdo it, this is something you shouldn't treat yourself.

For whatever reason, if your ovaries are not functioning optimally, you won't be able to adequately convert DHEA to the other hormones further down the pathway. When that happens, women tend to have the "excess androgen" side effects I showed in the chart for testosterone excess. Too much DHEA can cause exactly the same side effects as too much testosterone.

In addition, neuroendocrine research has found that women's testosterone receptors need to be "primed" with estradiol in order for the androgens to have optimal effects. So if you are given DHEA, but your estradiol levels are too low, you again have the risk of adverse side effects as well as increased irritability and restless sleep seen with excess testosterone.

In FMS and Chronic Fatigue, the issue is even more problematic: women tend to experience *worsening* muscle pain and spasm if the androgens (either DHEA or testosterone) are replaced *prior to* having optimal estradiol.

I have evaluated many fibromyalgia and fatigue patients who had been treated by other physicians with 50 to 100 mg of DHEA daily, and yet never checked estradiol levels or replaced estradiol when it was seriously low. All of the women I have seen who were treated with androgens alone had an *increase* muscle pain and spasm, particularly the muscles of the neck, scalp and back. In addition, the high doses of DHEA and low estradiol caused marked insomnia and restless sleep. These women then needed more of the muscle relaxant and sleep medications that in turn made them more tired during the day. The progression of their symptoms had become a vicious cycle—more androgens to treat fatigue, more muscle pain and restless sleep, then more medication to treat the sleep and pain, following by more daytime fatigue.

For women, it is really critical to first get the foundation of estradiol restored to optimal levels, and then add appropriate androgens in doses that keep the blood levels in healthy, physiologically natural ranges for women. It is a balancing act, as I continue to emphasize throughout my writings. Remember your basic body chemistry is different from a man's…you need a *woman's* balance restored.

Promises and Potential for the Future

Now that I have pointed out some of the "pitfalls" to watch for, what about promises for DHEA? DHEA has been promoted as the "feel-good" hormone, improving one's sense of well-being, energy, memory, and mental sharpness. We also hear claims that DHEA sparks an increase in sex drive, muscles and bone and can improve immune function. So what do the controlled studies actually show? Let's review some of these.

DHEA and Cognitive Function

Many marketing claims are made saying DHEA is the superhormone for improved brain function. Unfortunately, the few carefully done, placebo-controlled studies looking for cognitive benefits of DHEA have been disappointing. At least four double-blind placebo-controlled studies have been published in recent years that failed to find statistically significant evidence of DHEA having a positive effect on several measures of memory, attention or cognitive function. Six cross-sectional and six longitudinal studies found no clear evidence of DHEA having a beneficial effect on cognitive function or sense of well-being in men or women. Only one short two-week study by Wolf and colleagues showed improvement in immediate and delayed recall in women, but not in men. But in the same study, they tested four other cognitive measures and found

Remember

The correct balance of DHEA with estradiol and testosterone can be beneficial.

But you need reliable tests to check all of these hormones.

no other cognitive benefits on any of these tests. Dr. Wolf's group did several other clinical trials of DHEA using multiple outcome measures, and none of these showed any significant benefit of the hormone over placebo in men or women. The researchers considered that the brief improvement seen in recall in women in the one study was possibly due to chance, or might be an initial effect of DHEA being converted to estradiol or testosterone in the brain.

Reality:

Taking DHEA won't make you a genius.

Studies of Alzheimer's patients show that they commonly have low levels of DHEA, but this association is also found in many other conditions, so it isn't specific to Alzheimer's. No one yet knows whether the low DHEA helps contribute to the development of Alzheimers, or whether the disease causes effects in the brain that result in decreased brain and adrenal production of DHEA.

Dr. Hillen and colleagues published a study in 2000 that found that DHEA-S levels were lower in people followed over time who later developed Alzheimer's compared to those who did not. We also have research that shows loss of estradiol and testosterone can cause damage in the brain similar to that seen in Alzheimer's Disease. Loss of optimal thyroid hormone, and *excess* free cortisol, can both accelerate damage to cognitive function and increase the risk of Alzheimers, as well as effect DHEA levels, so it is hard to know which came first, the disease or the low hormone levels.

DHEA and Mood

Many manufactures of DHEA products claims that it helps depression, but again the results from controlled studies are mixed. There are some showing *high* DHEA-S levels are associated with depressive symptoms in premenopausal women, such as those with PCOS. There are others showing DHEA supplementation has reduced depressive symptoms in patients with major depression, Addison's Disease and HIV disease.

But these studies did not also look at the role of other hormones—estradiol, testosterone, and thyroid—and their effects on mood to see if the same benefits may have also occurred with supplementing these hormones. At this point, there are too many unanswered questions to be able to recommend people take DHEA instead of other, more proven approaches to help depression.

DHEA and Bone

Some clinicians have proposed that DHEA may help prevent osteoporosis, but again, we don't have good data on a bone-preserving effect from using DHEA. Dr. Casson's group studied DHEA replacement effects on various well-accepted markers of bone health, and found no change in urinary hydroxyproline, hydroxylysine, or collagen crosslink excretion, and no improvement in bone mineral density on DEXA testing at six months. Other studies have been similar in finding no consistent effect of DHEA to improve bone. There is one study, however, of women over age 60 who showed an increase in bone mineral density when given 50 mg of DHEA for a year, but this effect was not seen in the men in the study. Again, it isn't clear whether this improvement in bone density could have also been achieved with estradiol and/or testosterone supplementation.

DHEA and Immune Function

Evidence to date does not support DHEA being given routinely to healthy menopausal women for hormone replacement, but there are some situations in which DHEA does appear to have an important role. One of those is Systemic Lupus Erythematosis. Studies at UCLA using DHEA replacement for Lupus have been promising in reducing pain and other manifestations of the disease. Unfortunately, at the high doses (100 to 200 mg daily) used in the studies, many of the women developed significant unwanted side effects (facial hair, acne, irritability, for example), which limited their abil-

Caution:

There are too many unanswered questions to be able to recommend people take DHEA instead of other, more proven approaches to help depression.

ity to use it long term. It may be that future studies will show that lower doses maintain the benefits without causing so many negative side effects.

But if we consider the claims that DHEA improves immune function in older people across the board, I think it is important to note: None of the controlled studies of DHEA given to healthy older men and women found any particular immune system benefits if they simply had age-related low levels of DHEA but did not have specific medical disorders (Addison's, SLE, etc.).

DHEA and Sex Drive

Caution:

So far, current studies using DHEA are inconclusive.

The good news here is that there is one study of women age 70-79 who showed improved sexual interest, sexual arousal and sexual satisfaction after taking 50 mg of DHEA daily compared to placebo. These positive effects did not appear in younger women or earlier than the 6th month of a 12 month study, however, and the researchers felt that the benefits were more likely related to the rise in both estradiol and testosterone seen in the group taking DHEA.

The bad news is that men and younger women in the same study had no improvement in any of the sexual measures. In fact, for the men in this study taking DHEA, there was an increase in estradiol and no increase in testosterone, not exactly the effect they were looking for!

In all other age groups of men and women studied so far in placebo-controlled trials, there have not been any statistically significant improvements in sexual desire or arousal using DHEA alone. As I mentioned earlier, women in some of these studies not only had unwanted androgenic side effects, but they also had a decrease in their "good" HDL cholesterol, not a positive result.

DHEA and Fertility Treatment

Dr. Casson and his group have published results of a study giving DHEA to five healthy, non-smoking women less than 41 years of age who had a history of poor ovarian response to gonadotrophin stimulation during fertility treatment. All of the women in their study had Day 3 FSH levels of less than 20 mIU/ml. They hypothesized that DHEA might act to enhance the effect of insulin-like growth factor-1 and thereby improve ovarian hormone response to gonadotrophins. They found that giving 80 mg of DHEA daily for two months in this small number of patients led to higher levels of DHEA-S, testosterone and estradiol after the gonadotrophins were given.

They concluded from these results that for some women who have been poor responders, DHEA may possibly improve ovulation induction response, if they still have a normal FSH. This is an area of promising research that the investigators feel bears more study. I think it is important to note that the DHEA used in Dr. Casson's studies is prescription grade DHEA, formulated into tablets by Belmar Pharmacy in Lakewood, Colorado. As I mentioned earlier, over-the-counter DHEA is not the same level of quality or dose standardization as what reputable researchers use in their studies.

Caution:

Using DHEA can lead to some strange side effects.

Really... do you want more chin hair?

DHEA in Addison's Disease and Hypopituitarism

Addison's Disease, or Adrenal Insufficiency (A.I.), is an uncommon but very serious medical disorder in which DHEA use has been studied. True Addison's disease is rare. You should be properly diagnosed with appropriate medical tests before just accepting some-one telling you that you have "adrenal exhaustion" or adrenal insufficiency" based on a saliva test and then started on Cortef or other cortisone-type medicine. Taking corticosteroids when you don't really need them can cause other problems, and may mask a different underlying cause of your symptoms.

True Addison's Adrenal Insufficiency causes **marked weight loss** in all patients with the disease, so if you are *gaining* weight or haven't lost a great deal of weight, it's not likely that you have AI.

Other physical signs that could suggest Addison's disease include hair loss over the entire body but especially loss of axillary and pubic hair, loss of muscle, increased splotchy skin pigmentation, significantly low blood pressure, electrolyte imbalances, and an 8 AM cortisol less than 5-7 µg/dl.

If an 8 AM serum cortisol is greater than 10 µg/dl, true AI is again very unlikely, and you should be checked for other hormone imbalances causing similar symptoms. Endocrinologists are generally the best type of physician to see for an evaluation if you suspect you may have Addison's disease. Left untreated, Addisons' disease can be fatal.

When there is a true deficiency of adrenal function, all hormones produced by the adrenal gland are too low, making replacement therapy with corticosteroids necessary.

Replacing DHEA in Addison's Disease

More recently, researchers began to consider whether it is important to also replace the lost adrenal androgens, in particular DHEA. Women with adrenal insufficiency due to hypoactivity of the pituitary, also have loss of ovarian and thyroid hormone production, so they will have even more marked symptoms from the combination of androgen, estrogen and thyroid deficiency. This is another group of women who have been studied to determine whether DHEA offers benefits.

Professor Arit and colleagues in Germany used DHEA supplements in 24 women with documented Addison's disease to determine the effects on sexuality and well-being. Results were published in 1999 in the *New England Journal of Medicine*, and were promising.

Fourteen of the women had a primary form of adrenal insufficiency, and all were taking corticosteroid replacement medications. In this group, there were 17 women who were either hypogonadal (low estradiol and testosterone) or postmenopausal and 13 of these women were also taking some form of estrogen-progestin therapy. The women were given either 50 mg of DHEA or placebo for four weeks, and then crossed over to the opposite treatment to compare responses. The women were not told whether they were receiving the DHEA or the placebo pills.

Professor Arit's group found that supplemental DHEA produced increases in serum DHEA, DHEA-S and testosterone but no increase in estradiol levels. Sex hormone binding globulin (SHBG) was *decreased,* which mean that more of the sex hormones were available in the bloodstream in the free, active form. Total cholesterol was decreased, but an unwanted finding was that the good cholesterol (HDL) was also decreased with the DHEA therapy. There was significant improvement in overall well-being, depression, anxiety, sexual thoughts, sexual interest, and sexual satisfaction on several objective measures, as well as in the women's self-reports.

WISDOM:

Watch for the signs of androgen excess with OTC DHEA

Side effects that occurred were the well-known ones of excess androgen: acne, oily skin, increased body/facial hair, and loss of scalp hair (alopecia) during the time of active DHEA treatment. Decreasing the dose of DHEA helped to minimize or eliminate these unwanted side effects. The researchers concluded that DHEA was an appropriate therapeutic option for women with well-documented and properly diagnosed Addison's Disease.

Women who are taking chronic corticosteroid medications for a medical condition such as asthma, arthritis, allergies, or autoimmune disorders like Lupus typically experience symptoms from the way that these medications suppress ovarian and adrenal hormone production. People taking daily corticosteroids for medical conditions is actually a much more common problem than true Addison's disease. Women who have to take daily corticosteroids, such as prednisone and others, may benefit from low dose DHEA supplementation *if properly balanced with estradiol*. But there are not yet many studies to confirm that DHEA is beneficial in this situation, and there may actually be better improvements in energy, mood, muscle mass, bone and sex drive if women are given physiologically natural amounts of estradiol with testosterone instead of DHEA.

Summary

Drs. Katz and Morales from the University of California at San Diego summarized the current situation well:

"There is much international and multidisciplinary interest in the physiology and use of DHEA 'replacement' in men and menopausal women. The scientific community anxiously awaits the results of these investigations, but in the interim DHEA and/or DHEA-Sulfate (DHEAS) supplementation is not recommended as a therapeutic option in menopause outside of clinical trials."

I have seen too many complications of unregulated DHEA use in patients I have evaluated, particularly when women are given doses higher than 10-20 mg a day in the absence of adequate estradiol.

DHEA can be a double-edge sword for women, causing potentially serious problems when used over a long period of time. The weight gain, sweet cravings, acne, loss of scalp hair, irritability, insomnia, and muscle pain has been both disturbing, not to mention somewhat frightening, to these women.

Before you add DHEA or Cortef or other hormones, however, you need to be properly evaluated by a physician who is experienced in adrenal disorders and uses the medically-accepted diagnostic tests to check for adrenal problems.

Taking corticosteroid medications daily will suppress the adrenal and ovarian production of all your hormones, including DHEA, leading to symptoms similar to those seen in Addison's disease.

If you still feel that DHEA is something you want added to your hormone "recipe," I encourage you to first have

---

Wisdom:

Hormones levels fluctuate during the day.

It's usually best to check levels in the morning.

a thorough evaluation by your physician to have the appropriate blood tests done for all hormone levels, fasting glucose, lipids, and liver function.

Don't just have a saliva test for DHEA and make your decision on only one piece of the picture. If your DHEA levels are significantly decreased, and you have some of the symptoms that have been shown to be helped by DHEA, I suggest that you avoid over-the-counter products of unknown quality, and work with your physician to find a reputable compounding pharmacist who uses prescription grade DHEA to make tablets of known dose and quality.

Over-the-counter DHEA products are from *food-grade* sources, not the *pharmaceutical* (or prescription) *grade* DHEA used in research studies. Not all over-the-counter products deliver the amount they state on the label, and many products contain excessive doses for women's needs. Since there is the potential for marked adverse side effects of excess DHEA, as well as increased risks of long term health problems, make sure that your estradiol foundation is optimal before you add androgens like DHEA.

Then, if you start DHEA, make sure your physician re-checks your serum levels of hormones, fasting lipids, fasting glucose, and liver function at appropriate intervals. You should also pay attention to what is happening to the quality of your sleep and your scalp hair if you are taking DHEA—both of these can be adversely affected if you are taking too much. If you start taking DHEA and are gaining weight around the middle of your body or you start craving sweets, these are other clues that you should talk with your physician and may need to cut back on the dose.

As with all androgens, DHEA should be started in low doses and increased slowly, making sure that you also have a foundation of optimal estradiol to help prevent unwanted side effects or health problems.

Caveat:

Don't be misled by practitioners who tell you that you have "adrenal insufficiency" based on saliva or hair tests.

These tests are not reliable.

Dr. Vliet's memonics to guide you:

Don't forget…
Hormones, including DHEA
Effect
All of you!

If that doesn't help, try this one:

Don't forget, *women's*
Hormone balance means
Estradiol *first*,
Androgen *after*…

Caution:

What you
don't know
can hurt you.

Especially
when it
comes
to taking
powerful
hormones.

Chapter 8

The Testosterone Revolution for Women: Restoring Your Sexuality, Energy and Vitality

Bioidentical Testosterone

Through the miracle of the laboratory, *soy*beans are turned into *boy*beans to give you testosterone that is an exact molecular replica of the human molecule made by the ovary. Our body does not have the enzymes to do this conversion simply by eating soy foods, so the changes have to be made in the laboratory. Then the bioidentical testosterone is *micronized*, or made into tiny particles just as bioidentical estradiol and progesterone are, so they can be made into tablets or capsules to be taken orally and not be completely lost to digestion.

FACT:

Soybeans are not the answer you have been led to believe.

U.S.P. prescription grade micronized testosterone is standardized, and when I request a compounding pharmacist to make a prescription for one of my patients, I know exactly how much of the hormone that preparation will have in it. I can fine-tune the amount for each individual, based on symptoms and follow-up tests. Testosterone U.S.P. can also be made up in a variety of *non-oral* ways to take it: sublingual troches, creams, gels, patches, pellets, suppositories, injections... and even nasal sprays!

Lots of exciting new product options are "in the pipeline" in clinical trials. The studies are on track to be submitted to the FDA for review, evaluation and hopefully approval, possibly as early as 2006. I describe later in this chapter some of these new products being developed in doses suitable for women.

In the meantime, how can women get bioidentical testosterone? Until the commercial products are approved and available, all of the various ways to take testosterone can be made to individual prescriptions by compounding pharmacists, based on a physician's prescription. All compounding pharmacists have access to the same raw powder of U.S.P. pharmaceutical grade micronized testosterone.

Wisdom:

Synthetic bioidentical hormones are "natural" but not all "natural" hormones are bioidentical to human ones.

The major difference lies in what formula each particular pharmacist uses in making up the compounded prescriptions. These compounded preparations can vary a great deal depending on the particular formula used and what binders the pharmacist puts in the preparation.

This is quite different from standardized FDA-approved commercial medications that are the same whether you buy them at Costco or your friendly local drugstore.

Pills, Potions, Lotions, or Shots?

There are many ways to deliver hormones to the body. Various delivery systems can make an enormous difference in how the hormones affect you. Swallow a pill? Use a cream? Have an injection? What about vaginal forms?

The method chosen determines what dose is appropriate, the amount that is absorbed, how it is metabolized or changed into other forms, what effects—desirable or undesirable occur, what the side effects might be, and what the particular risks could be.

Keep in mind, each woman is different, and her needs can also change over time. So what works for you now may need to be modified in years to come. What works for your friend may *not* work for you.

There are advantages and disadvantages of each delivery method, especially when we are dealing with the ovarian hormones. Let's look at what they are.

When you take any medicine by mouth and <u>swallow</u> it (as opposed to letting it dissolve under your tongue, called *sublingual* delivery), it has to undergo what we call the "first-pass" metabolism in the liver. This first step changes hormones that dissolve better in fat into compounds that can be absorbed and carried by the watery bloodstream to the rest of the body. Sometimes this first step in the liver creates compounds that are useful and helpful, and sometimes the hepatic first pass metabolism creates compounds that have unwanted side effects for some people.

Progesterone is one good example of what a difference the route of delivery can make. When this hormone is taken in pill form and swallowed, it is converted in the liver to compounds we call *metabolites* that are chemically different from progesterone. These new metabolites have very potent sedative and depressant effects on the brain, even more potent than the short-acting barbiturate *methohexital* that dentists have used to put people to sleep when having teeth pulled.

Vaginal progesterone is absorbed directly into the bloodstream and bypasses the "first pass" change in the liver, so it isn't changed into all these sedative compounds and women don't feel as lethargic, depressed, or "uncontrollably sleepy during the day," a description I often hear from women who take progesterone in pill form.

All the non-oral forms of estradiol and testosterone are absorbed directly into the bloodstream as the hormone itself and bypass the "first pass" liver changes into new compounds. Non-oral delivery is more similar to the way the ovary releases hormones directly into the bloodstream. There are many advantages to non-oral delivery. I summarized those in the chart that follows.

Fact:

How you take a hormone is as important as how much you take.

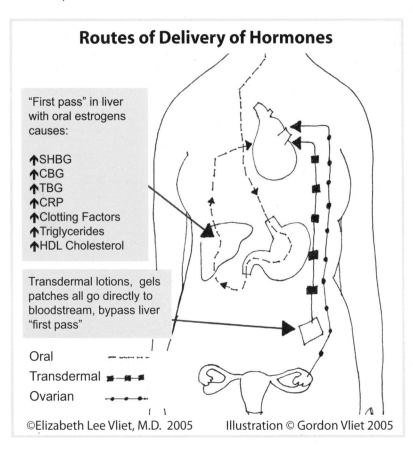

Routes of Delivery of Hormones

"First pass" in liver
with oral estrogens
causes:

↑SHBG
↑CBG
↑TBG
↑CRP
↑Clotting Factors
↑Triglycerides
↑HDL Cholesterol

Transdermal lotions, gels
patches all go directly to
bloodstream, bypass liver
"first pass"

Oral   — · — · —

Transdermal   ▪—▪—▪

Ovarian   · — · — ·

©Elizabeth Lee Vliet, M.D. 2005   Illustration © Gordon Vliet 2005

Advantages of NON-Oral Testo Delivery

The most "natural" way to restore testosterone or estradiol is by
non-oral options, such as a slowly absorbed cream, or a patch when
that is available. Non-oral forms have advantages because:

- ☙ Bypasses the liver on first pass–in other words, doesn't break
  down into other compounds that may have ill effects

- ☙ Doesn't increase the "bad" cholesterol or lower the "good"
  cholesterol, helps lower blood pressure

- ☙ Keeps levels steady in normal range, avoiding unwanted
  highs or lows, which helps prevent headaches

- ☙ Minimizes undesirable side effects and liver interactions with
  other medications

©Elizabeth Lee Vliet, M.D. 2005

Oral Tablets and Capsules

In addition to individually compounded bioidentical testosterone, FDA-approved products, Estratest and Estratest H.S., are available as fixed dose tablets of *esterified estrogens* (EE), which are similar to Premarin, and *methyl testosterone* (MT), a more potent form of testosterone. Since it only comes in two strengths, Estratest doesn't allow flexibility in dosing to meet your individual needs. Estratest has been the only commercial option available for women in the United States and it has been widely used for women who have had their ovaries removed during hysterectomy, as well as for naturally menopausal women.

Studies by Sherwin, Gelfand, Sarrel, Notelovitz, and others have found that women using Estratest after hysterectomy or during natural menopause have much better effects on sex drive than women using estrogen alone. This certainly makes sense with our understanding of testosterone effects on sexual arousal in women. These studies have typically compared oral estrogen with oral estrogen and testosterone in Estratest.

Remember that oral estrogens, especially esterified or horse-derived mixtures, cause the liver to make much more SHBG. Then the excess SHBG attaches to the free testosterone, making it inactive. Women who use a non-oral form of estradiol don't have this extra stimulation of SHBG, and will have higher levels of free testosterone, even if the total testosterone has declined somewhat. Non-oral estradiol is less likely to cause low libido since more testosterone is available in the active form.

Testosterone in the oral form, however, can sometimes cause a *decrease* in the "good" HDL and an increase in total and LDL ("bad") cholesterol because of the first pass effects in the liver. Oral testosterone is also more likely to raise blood pressure than is non-oral testosterone, again due to effects from the liver first pass metabolism. For women who already have high blood pressure, or high cholesterol with high LDL

Wisdom:

Non-oral estradiol is less likely to lower free testosterone ... and your libido!

and low HDL, it really is important to consider using testosterone in one of the non-oral ways.

I described additional problems in Chapter 6 that I have encountered in patients using Estratest: it doesn't provide very much of the 17-beta estradiol women lose at menopause and it gives high amounts of estrone, the estrogen made by fat tissue after menopause. As I noted, methyl testosterone is more potent than bioidentical testosterone. This potency difference can mean that the dose in Estratest, or even it's half-strength form, is too much for some women.

Caution:

For some women, Estratest is too much methyl testosterone and not enough estradiol.

Josie's Story

Josie had a hysterectomy and removal of her ovaries in her early forties because of endometriosis. Her gynecologist initially started her on Premarin, but it caused her to have migraines and increased blood pressure. Then he tried Estratest to see if this would relieve her headaches and improve her libido. By the time I saw her for a consult about a year later, she had completely lost her soprano voice.

For some women, this wouldn't have been a serious problem but Josie is a professional *soprano* opera singer. She could no longer perform in concerts, and was on the verge of losing the career she loved, plus her main source of income. Needless to say, she was extremely distressed by this.

She had also gained a great deal of weight, in spite of careful attention to a healthy meal plan, and her blood pressure had skyrocketed. She had begun having frequent migraine headaches, although she had never had these before she began Premarin after her hysterectomy.

Her hormone evaluation told an interesting story, as I almost always find. Her estradiol was too low at less than 30 pg/ml, while her total testosterone was significantly elevated at 176 ng/dl. Her free testosterone level, another important measure, was also markedly elevated.

It was obvious to me why her voice had deepened so

much. This is a well-described side effect of excess testosterone in women.

Too much testosterone can make you ravenously hungry, so it is hard to control your weight. High testosterone, especially if estradiol is low, can cause high blood pressure and headaches. These hormone imbalances clearly explained the multiple changes she had experienced in her voice and body.

I recommended she stop the Estratest, and use a transdermal estradiol patch for better absorption. Non-oral estradiol also causes more dilation of blood vessels, thereby helping to lower blood pressure. A patch provides more stable estradiol delivery that helps prevent hormone swings that can trigger migraines.

Wisdom:

Fixed dose combination products can make it hard to individualize hormone therapy.

Since her testosterone was too high, I suggested she just stop Estratest and let the levels fall gradually. I explained that she could take bioidentical micronized testosterone separately once her estradiol was optimal. My goal was to help her adjust the testosterone so it was enough to improve her libido and energy level, but not adversely affect her voice, weight or blood pressure.

At her follow up appointment three months later, she was exuberant.

> "I feel so much better now! My voice is completely clear and back to normal. I am so grateful that my vocal cords weren't permanently damaged by all that testosterone. My headaches are much less frequent now, and my blood pressure is back to normal."

At this appointment, her estradiol was in the optimal range of 120 pg/ml, and her testosterone had come down to 13 ng/dl, quite a dramatic change from two months earlier on Estratest. With her level this low, and her libido "gone to zero," I gave her a prescription for a very low dose testosterone cream to use several times a week. Six months later, she was doing very well on her new hormone regimen, her migraines had not come back, her voice was fine, and she headed off to Italy for a series of concerts.

A year later at her next appointment, she said,

> "We got the voice fixed and I am really pleased with that part. I haven't had a migraine headache in over a year since the change to the patch. My primary care physician was very good and agreed to work with all the things I learned from you."

She was now using one Climara transdermal estradiol patch every 5 days, and occasionally added another patch when she was under a lot of stress and seemed to be metabolizing the estradiol faster. She used the testosterone cream occasionally when she wanted to have better sexual arousal, but decided not to use it daily because she did not want to risk negative effects on her voice again.

Since she had had a hysterectomy, she did not need progesterone. This was fortunate since progesterone would also have adversely affected her vocal cords. She was quite happy with her current hormone "recipe," and thankful that she could continue the singing career she loved.

Creams and Patches

Josie's story leads us to the benefits of creams and other non-oral forms of testosterone. Testosterone used in a non-oral form such as a cream, patch, pellet, or injection doesn't have the same degree of negative impact on the cholesterol profile or blood pressure that we see with oral testosterone.

The Intrinsa patch now in clinical trials showed this important difference in effect on cholesterol with transdermal testosterone bypassing the liver. Published data from the clinical trials to date show no significant difference between placebo and the testosterone patch on lipids, blood pressure, or weight. The testosterone patch also gives much more stable blood levels over time than the creams and gels, which for women like Josie, can help reduce the tendency for hormone swings to trigger headaches.

Since the testosterone patch isn't yet available in the United States, the compounded cream gave me the suitable alternative that would allow Josie to control how much and how often she used it. Like the patch, a cream that is more slowly absorbed than a gel is also less likely to cause headaches from a rapid rise in blood level that can happen with oral forms, *IF* the non-oral dose is kept in the natural physiologic range for women.

Gels and Troches

Sublingual troches and alcohol-based gels are often touted as "best," but this isn't always the case. For some women, gels and troches are absorbed so fast and cause such a rapid rise in blood level of testosterone that they feel anxious, agitated, aggressive, and irritable or may have pounding headaches, palpitations, racing heartbeat, or insomnia.

Wisdom:

You may prefer an approach *you* can control more easily.

I tried a compounded testosterone gel after my hysterectomy some years ago and it hit me so fast and so dramatically, I thought my head would explode. I felt like I could kill a gorilla barehanded! I have been keenly aware ever since just what my patients mean when they say "The testosterone is too much all at once."

I have seen many women, and even some men, who had similar reactions to both testosterone or estradiol gels. You need to be aware that speed of absorption can be good, or can be quite bad, depending on how your particular body responds. A *rapid* rise in blood level of testosterone can cause unpleasant symptoms not only when the level is rising, but also when it wears off too fast. You can feel a "crash," with depressed or lethargic feelings when testosterone falls too fast. Generally, I prefer the slower absorption and delivery forms like patches and creams that are designed to be more slowly absorbed.

Injectables

There are a number of injectable testosterone preparations, but not all of these are the bioidentical form of testosterone. Some are the potent synthetic preparations that even at low doses may cause unwanted androgenic effects in women. Most of the commercially available injectable forms of testosterone have been made in doses that are for men. This makes it hard to achieve the right dose and optimal results for women, which is another reason testosterone has gotten a bad reputation for having so many unwanted side effects.

Even if the dose is low enough for women, there is another pitfall to watch out for when using injectable forms. Shots of testosterone often give high levels at the beginning and wear off rather unpredictably, at times making you feel like you are on a hormonal roller coaster. Many women tell me they don't like this effect of too much stimulation right after the injection, and then having to deal with the "lows" that occur when it wears off. How can you feel like you are on an "even keel" to get through your day if you are having such a rise and fall in testosterone?

Caution:

Pellets and implants can be more difficult for you to control.

Pellets and Implants

Testosterone *pellets* are available also. These are sometimes called *implants*, since they are surgically inserted under the skin in the fat pads on the hip. Pellets and implants are not FDA-approved commercial products, so they have to be prepared to individual prescription. They can be formulated to give a lower dose and more gradual absorption than the injectable forms, but the pellets also wear off unpredictably, and make it harder to keep you feeling "even" without getting too much at the beginning and too little at the end. Some women really like the pellets, others have had very bad experiences with them.

I prefer not to use pellets (implants) because I want to use methods that the *woman herself can easily control*, based on how she is feeling. With pills or creams (or patches when available), each woman decides whether to use it that day. With the implants, you have to go to the doctor's office and have them surgically placed under the skin. Then you are stuck with them until either you go back to the doctor and have the pellet taken out or until it wears off. Injections have the same problem—once it's done, if you have any bad side effects, you have to wait until the dose wears off. You can't take back an injection. I occasionally do prescriptions for injectable testosterone, but I use very low doses and have patients start with a very tiny amount in the syringe, maybe only 0.1 ml, until we can see how she responds.

Overall, I prefer to use hormone preparations that give *you* more flexibility with the amount you use and when you need to change a patch or take a pill, so that you have more control over *your* hormone management.

Topical preparations for the vagina and vulva

Gynecologists have used topical vaginal testosterone ointments and creams, especially to treat lichen sclerosus, as I mentioned in Chapter 4. The type of base and dose are the main differences between these preparations and those designed to use on the abdomen or inner thigh. Vaginal and vulvar tissues have a very good blood supply, and the skin is thinner and has less fat underneath than on the abdomen or thigh. Consequently, testosterone is rapidly absorbed from the vulva or vaginal application. This means a *topical* preparation to strengthen and heal vaginal or vulvar tissue needs to be a much smaller dose than what would be given for *systemic* effects throughout the total body.

Some physicians and authors recommend putting testosterone in a petrolatum ointment. Keep in mind that "petrolatum" is a petroleum-based product and can be very irritating to sensitive tissues. Mineral oil bases can also cause more drying of tissue that may already be too dry and painful.

I prefer to use a hypo-allergenic base less likely to further irritate inflamed tissues. If you are having more irritation with something the doctor prescribed to help treat itching, burning, and dryness, it's usually not due to the hormone itself. Ask your health professional to change your prescription to a hypoallergenic cream without mineral oil, preservatives or petroleum derivatives.

Caution:

Use much lower doses for vulva and vaginal use... they are very well-absorbed.

Caution:

Petroleum derived bases for ointments can be very irritating to sensitive tissues.

New Products in the Pipeline...

There has been a great deal more interest in products to help women's sexual difficulties, possibly as an outgrowth of the interest in sexual function fueled by the development of Viagra and similar products for men. We now have several pharmaceutical companies developing testosterone preparations in doses designed for *women's* bodies and using *bioidentical* testosterone instead of *methyl* testosterone.

What lies ahead?

Androsorb
Intrinsa
Libigel
Tostrelle
and
others

Procter and Gamble, in partnership with Watson Pharmaceuticals, developed the first patch for women, called *Intrinsa.* The clinical trial studies have been completed and the data published for surgically menopausal women, and for another group of naturally menopausal women. In both groups, the Intrinsa testosterone patch resulted in significant increases in sexual desire and sexually satisfying experiences when compared to placebo, and there were very few side effects reported.

Intrinsa was initially "fast-tracked" by the FDA to be considered for approval in 2005. Sadly for women waiting for the patch, at the Advisory Committee meeting on December 2, 2004, members of the committee wanted additional safety data over a longer period of time. At this point, no one knows when the Intrinsa approval process could be restarted and when we might have it available to women. Clinical trials are continuing, however, so I am hopeful we will have the testosterone patch approved for the treatment of low sexual desire before too many more years go by. I personally hope that in addition to the data on sexual function, we will see more studies showing all the *other* documented effects of testosterone on brain function, muscle strength, energy level, and mood.

Several smaller biotech pharmaceutical companies have also begun developing other forms of testosterone delivery systems. In 2005, BioSante has a testosterone gel, called *LibiGel,* in phase III clinical trials, while Cellegy is in phase III testing of its testosterone gel,

Tostrelle. Columbia Labs has completed phase I studies of a testosterone vaginal gel, and Novavax has a testosterone cream called *Androsorb* in phase II studies. Vivus is in phase II testing of a measured dose testosterone nasal spray.

I have seen reports in business magazines that there are talks between Noven Pharmaceuticals, and Procter and Gamble about developing a combined testosterone-estradiol transdermal patch. This could certainly simplify things, and would mean you wouldn't have to have patches all over your tummy! Noven already makes Vivelle DOT, a highly successful estradiol patch and a estradiol-progestin patch called Combi Patch. It should not be much more difficult to make a patch that contains either estradiol and testosterone for women who have had a hysterectomy, or even a patch with all three hormones for women who still have a uterus and need the progestin.

So, if you feel your libido has gone for good, don't give up yet. There is hope on the horizon that in the not-too-distant future, you may have an FDA-approved commercial, standardized product that is even covered by your prescription plan! In the meantime, we can still use individually compounded testosterone preparations to successfully help women who have lost this critical hormone.

Wisdom:

Commercial products in development may not have this same problem, since they use polymer technology, not available for compounding individual prescriptions.

Dosing Issues

Currently, commercial brands of testosterone don't have doses low enough for women on a daily basis. Compounded prescriptions allow us to use lower doses and fine-tune what each individual needs until we have additional FDA-approved options. I often recommend a sustained release tablet or capsule, or a slow-release cream form. Oral doses generally are 1- 4 mg daily.

Doses for all non-oral forms (transdermal cream, vaginal and sublingual) need to be much lower than oral ones. The non-oral forms are more rapidly and

Fact

2% creams contain too much testosterone for women.

completely absorbed since they don't go through the first pass metabolic breakdown in the liver. This is a crucial point. You and your health professionals need to understand this, because many women get excessive doses of testosterone creams or sublingual troches, which can create horrible side effects.

Most women need only very small amounts of testosterone to achieve desired benefits. For example, as I mentioned in Chapter 6, a 2% testosterone cream (widely recommended in a number of women's health books) contains **20 mg/gram** of cream delivering about **20 times** the dose most women need in this readily absorbed form. A 1% cream can contain 10 mg per gram of cream, and 10 mg a day is still too much for women. These creams are typically very well absorbed, and can quickly give testosterone levels in the healthy *male* range.

Wisdom:

Non-oral doses should usually be only 1/10th of a typical *oral* dose.

By comparison, most of my testosterone prescriptions are in the range of 0.1mg/gm up to sometimes 1 mg/gm (0.1%) of cream (1 gram = ¼ teaspoon of cream). I start patients on 1.00 – 1.25 mg of oral sustained release micronized testosterone, and gradually increase based on the woman's description of symptoms and her serum levels. I find that most of my patients achieve the desirable response with an oral testosterone dose between 1 and 4 mg a day. Very rarely have I had to prescribe an oral dose more than that.

A safe rule of thumb for a starting point is that a cream form of the hormone should be about 1/10th of an oral dose. The amount should then be adjusted based on your response and your serum hormone levels.

I recommend that my patients re-check the testosterone level in the morning before a next dose, to be sure it isn't too high 24 hours after taking it. If I want to know the *peak* level, to be sure the level isn't getting too high soon after a dose, I request a blood level 4 hours after an oral dose, or 2-3 hours after a testosterone cream is applied.

Update on Testosterone and Breast Cancer Risk

Since the July 2002 announcement that the estrogen-progestin group of the WHI was being stopped due to increased health risks, many women have been psychologically traumatized by the fear that taking hormones would increase their risk of breast cancer. Millions of women immediately, often without consultation with their physicians, stopped all hormones even though the study only used one type of hormone, Premarin with the synthetic progestin MPA.

Most women have not been given the information that using this combination estrogen-progestin product resulted in an actual degree of increased risk of breast cancer for an *individual* woman that was exceedingly small, only about 0.1% per year. Risk of dying in a car accident is certainly far greater, yet we still drive our cars to maintain our quality of life.

Keep in mind what I have discussed earlier: Premarin contains estrogens foreign to the human female body, and the dose of MPA given to the elderly women in the WHI was actually a greater amount of progestin than we use in young women for birth control pills. In my opinion, it isn't surprising that this product had so many adverse effects in older women.

The second arm of the WHI was stopped in 2004 when researchers began to see a higher risk of stroke in the older women in the study. This arm of the WHI was made up of women who had a hysterectomy and did not have to take the progestin. They were only taking Premarin. When the end of the study was announced, news stories focused on the stroke concerns.

They *did not* mention that the estrogen-only group had a slightly *lower risk of breast cancer* than the control group taking no hormones. Some news reports even referred to the first WHI group and often mistakenly claimed "estrogen" caused an increase in risk of breast

Caution:

What you hear or see on the nightly news isn't exactly the entire story.

It may be the easiest or most sensational to report.

cancer. Again, women became more frightened of hormones, and even more women abruptly stopped their therapy.

When the FDA considered the request for approval of the testosterone patch for women, they used the results of the WHI with estrogen-progestin to raise concerns about a possible increase in breast cancer with testosterone, and then gave this as a reason to withhold approval of patch.

With more women now aware that testosterone can help improve sex drive, and also has a host of other benefits, it becomes important to look at the question of the effects of testosterone on breast cancer risk. While it is a complicated picture, and still much that we don't know with certainty, there is encouraging news on the effect of adding testosterone to hormone therapy.

New Findings

Testosterone may be a natural "protector" for breast cell growth triggered by estrogen and progesterone in the menstrual cycle.

Let's explore what we know at this time

The normal ovary produces more testosterone than estrogens throughout our lives. During our menstrual cycle, breast cell proliferation, or growth, occurs in both the follicular (estrogen-dominant) phase and the luteal (progesterone dominant) phase. The most rapid growth, however, occurs under the influence of *progesterone* in the second half of our cycle each month. Both experimental and clinical data suggest that a normal balance of testosterone and other androgens provides an inhibitory, or blocking, effect on breast cell growth stimulated by our own estrogen and progesterone during our menstrual cycles, or during estrogen—progestin therapy.

A number of studies of hormone use in various populations of women, plus studies in Rheusus monkeys, as well as basic science studies of cellular effects of testosterone on breast tissue—all suggest that addition of testosterone to hormone therapy does not increase, and may indeed reduce, risk of breast cancer. Based on the collective findings from cell cultures, animal and human studies, researchers are beginning to think that testosterone may serve as a natural protector of the breast by inhibiting breast cell growth that occurs in the normal menstrual cycle human.

For example, Drs. Dimitrakakis, Zhou and Bondy at the National Institutes of Health (NIH) studied the effects of added ovarian hormones in natural dose ranges on growth (proliferation) of breast tissue in Rhesus monkeys that had their own ovaries removed. There were four groups: no hormones (control, or placebo group), estradiol (E2) alone, estradiol plus testosterone (E2 + T), and estradiol plus progesterone (E2 + P). All groups of animals had similar levels of estradiol. Both the E2 alone and E2 + P groups had about a three-fold increase in the index of breast cell proliferation when compared with the placebo group getting no hormones.

The good news was that the E2 + T group had *no increase in the proliferation index*, compared with the placebo group.

In further studies, Dr. Dimitrakakis' group used an androgen receptor blocker medication in normally cycling monkeys to show that there was *more breast cellular growth* in cycles when androgens were *blocked*. They found other changes in various chemical messengers and receptors that further suggested testosterone was having a physiological protective effect on the breast tissue in these primates.

From their series of studies, they concluded that testosterone, along with other androgens, normally inhibits growth of breast tissue stimulated by estrogen and progesterone during the menstrual cycle, or with estrogen-progestin therapy after menopause.

To add to the picture suggesting testosterone and other androgens do not increase the risk of breast cancer, evidence from a variety of cellular studies suggests that testosterone may lower the risk of breast cancer several ways: by changing the ratio of estrogen receptor alpha and beta in a positive direction, by altering

Interesting Note:

Evidence from a variety of cellular studies suggests that testosterone may lower the risk of breast cancer several ways various growth-promoting signaling systems in the breast, and by contributing to the natural cell death (*apoptosis*) that helps stop the uncontrolled growth that can lead to cancer.

There are a number of studies of women with PCOS who have high levels of androgens beginning in puberty. This group of women has not shown a significantly increased risk of breast cancer later in life, although they *do have an increased risk of endometrial cancer*. In fact, one 1991 study found a slightly less than expected risk of breast cancer in women with PCOS, but no one knows whether this is a cause—and—effect result of high androgens or due to some other factors.

Australian physicians at a specialty hormone therapy clinic in Adelaide have been using testosterone to supplement standard hormone therapy (HT) for about 25 years. They noticed that they rarely saw abnormal mammograms in women taking testosterone *with* standard estrogen-progestin therapy. They decided to do a systematic review of breast cancer incidence in their patient population. The results were quite interesting!

They used a baseline comparison group from South Australia taking no hormones, and compared this placebo group with:

> ❧ A group of their patients taking conjugated equine estrogens (CEE, or Premarin) and medroxyprogesterone acetate (MPA) but *no testosterone*

> ❧ A group of their patients taking CEE plus MPA *and testosterone*

> ❧ A group taking estrogen with testosterone

After a little over five years, they found that the women on all three hormones (E + P + T) had about the same number of cases of breast cancer as the control group on no hormones. But the women taking E+P *alone* had a 30% increase in breast cancer compared to controls.

This rate of increase in breast cancer in the E + P group was similar to the increase initially reported for the E + P group in the United States WHI study.

The Australian physicians noted that there was a fairly high rate of positive family history for breast cancer rates in their participants, which actually made the women at higher risk for developing the disease (28% and 30% positive family history for E + T and E + P + T, respectively). The authors felt that the likely reason they saw more patients with a positive family history of breast cancer was due that the referring primary care physicians did not feel comfortable prescribing any hormones for women with a positive family history.

Other possible risk factors were fairly similar for both hormone therapy groups, such as average age at menopause, number of children, length of time on hormone therapy (on estrogen for an average of about 8 years, and on the testosterone for between 5-6 years). The *addition of testosterone* was the primary difference between the groups that might account for the lower rate of breast cancers.

Rates Of Breast Cancer In Hormone Users And Non-users

	Breast Cancer Rate per 100,000 women	Author/Year	Yrs Followed
No hormone therapy (control population)	283	MWS	2.6 years
Estrogen/androgen	115	S. Australia	5.4 years
Estrogen/progestin and Androgen	293	S. Australia	5.9 years
Estrogen/progestin	380	WHI	5.2 years

MWS = Million Women Study, UK; WHI = Women's Health Initiative, US

Adding to the complexity of the picture, studies show differences in response to androgens depending on whether a woman is premenopausal or postmenopausal. For example, DHEA and androstenediol *stimulated* the growth of some forms of breast cancer cells in postmenopausal women, but these same androgens had an inhibitory effect on these same cancer cell types in younger, premenopausal women.

On the other hand, testosterone and DHT both *inhibited growth* of these same cancer cell lines, independent of the presence of estradiol. This inhibitory effect was lost when the cells were treated first with an androgen blocker, flutamide. There have also been clinical studies showing success with androgens in treating breast cancer, with a similar degree of success to that seen with tamoxifen.

So what's the bottom line? At this time, we don't have enough long term studies to be able to say with certainty that breast cancer risk is reduced by adding testosterone to menopausal hormone therapy or added for younger women with low androgen levels due to birth control pills or early ovarian decline. It will take a large-scale clinical trial of the size of the Women's Health Initiative to be able to answer such a question. In the current climate of fear about hormones, it may not be feasible to conduct such a study.

But in looking at all of the information we do have, a number of researchers are now suggesting that addition of testosterone to the usual estrogen-progestin menopause therapy may help to reduce breast proliferation that has been thought to increase breast cancer risk over time. Since there has been a fear that using testosterone therapy for women with sexual dysfunction may increase later risk of breast cancer, it is indeed encouraging to see so many clinical observations and experimental data to suggest that testosterone may actually have a *protective* effect on the breast.

Finding What's Right for You: Tracking Your Responses

I have talked in earlier chapters about the risks and adverse effects of too much testosterone, and some of those are also summarized in the chart that follows. There are several steps *you* can take to minimize your risks of unwanted effects from testosterone:

- Make a "self-check" list of the symptoms you feel will be helped by testosterone, based on what you have learned in this book.

- Make a "self-check" list of health risks, family history, or medical problems that you think may cause problems if you take testosterone and discuss these with your physician.

- Make sure you have a thorough metabolic laboratory evaluation, including fasting cholesterol profile and tests of liver and kidney function, as a baseline before deciding whether to try testosterone. Do follow up checks at regular intervals.

- Don't just start taking the prescription hormone or over-the-counter DHEA based on symptoms alone. I have suggested some of the important tests in the next chapter.

- Have a complete hormone profile and make sure you use the more reliable blood test methods to determine your hormone levels

- Have current physical exam, mammogram and Pap.

- Make sure your estradiol level is optimal before you add testosterone.

- Make sure you talk with your physician about herbs, supplements and other medicines you are taking that may interfere with testosterone.

TESTOSTERONE - BALANCE IS THE KEY

To help you make the important decisions about what is best for you and your health needs, I have summarized in the following table benefits of adding testosterone to a hormone therapy regimen. I have also given you some pointers on what to look for as effects of too little and too much testosterone, or DHEA. Most women need only very small amounts of testosterone for positive results.

DR. VLIET'S GUIDE TO TESTOSTERONE EFFECTS

TOO LITTLE	JUST RIGHT	TOO MUCH
low energy	normal energy	hyper feelings
loss of sex drive	normal libido	increased libido
slowed down, lethargic	alert, interested	"scattered" thoughts
decreased attention	normal attention	similar to A.D.D.
mild-to-moderate depressed mood, feeling "blah"	positive, upbeat	irritable, anxious, edgy, mood tense, aggressive
fewer dreams, loss of sexual dreams	normal dreams	intense dreaming, intense possibly violent dreams
excessive sleep, tired on awakening	normal sleep	restless, disrupted sleep
thinning and loss of scalp hair, pubic hair	hair thicker, grows normally	excess facial and body hair, scalp hair loss
dry, thin skin	normal skin	acne, oily skin
muscle aches, weakness	normal muscle tone/strength	muscle spasms, tenseness and pain

©Elizabeth Lee Vliet, MD 1995-2005

Chapter 9

The Savvy Woman's Testosterone ACTION Plan: Restoring Your Hormone Balance for Zest, Vitality…and Feeling Sexy Again!

Why bother with tests before you start on your hormones? Why not just go ahead and begin? Wouldn't that be easier, cheaper, and faster? Perhaps. But then, if you don't have the baseline tests, how do you really know the underlying *cause* of your symptoms? Are you low in estradiol only, or are both estradiol and testosterone too low? Is your thyroid out of whack? Is your cortisol too high causing similar symptoms? What's really going on? How do you know, if you don't get the proper tests? And how to you know where you need to be in terms of the amount you take? Wouldn't it be nice to have some clues about *why* you are having your current symptoms? Wouldn't it be helpful to know how your treatment is doing in meeting your goals?

Question:

How can you know where you need to be going… if you don't know where you *are*?

What can you do if your testosterone level is low? Your doctor can check blood levels of your ovarian hormones, and these are more reliable than other types of testing. Objective laboratory testing you to know *what's wrong,* and then allows you and your doctor to work together to find the combination of hormones and the right doses tailored to meet your unique needs.

What should you be looking for as a desirable target range for testosterone? In my clinical experience, if women have optimal levels of estradiol as a foundation, they typically experience their usual energy level and libido when serum (blood) levels of *total* testosterone are between 40 and 60 ng/dl. The serum free testosterone (serum) is typically about 1-2 percent of the total testosterone. I find that total testosterone levels below about 20 ng/dl are usually too low to maintain one's libido, and energy. The majority of women I have evaluated for loss of libido or severe fatigue have had total testosterone levels of less than 10-15 ng/dl. This is especially true if they had surgical removal of one or both ovaries, or had fertility treatments that deplete follicles and affect later hormone production. Such low levels of testosterone are certainly understandable factors that help explain fatigue, loss of muscle strength, and marked decrease in sexual desire.

Wisdom:

Testosterone occurs in the blood 3 ways: free, weakly-bound, and bound to SHBG

What Should Be Measured?

I explained in earlier chapters that testosterone is carried in the bloodstream three ways: free (the readily available, biologically active portion), *weakly bound* to albumin (still active, called *bioavailable*), and *tightly bound* to sex hormone binding globulin (making it inactive but available to move into the free, active portion). The most current research has shown that it is *not only* the *free* testosterone that is biologically active at the receptor sites. The portion that is *weakly bound* to serum albumin is also now known to be active at certain of the testosterone receptors. Serum (blood) assays measure all three of these circulating forms.

That's why I use the blood test regularly in my patients: it gives me a complete picture of the amount of testosterone you have that's readily available to act at tissues of the body, plus the total amount you have "in storage" that your body can call upon when needed. I also find that the ratio of total to free testosterone is important in helping me determine the amount needed, and the effects of other hormones on the testosterone balance. Imbalances between total and free testosterone give me clues as to what direction to take in making dose adjustments to help an individual woman improve the response or reduce side effects.

What about Saliva and Urine Hormone Tests?

You may have seen ads for testing your hormones with home kits using saliva or urine. There has been quite a consumer marketing campaign for these tests over the Internet, through pharmacies, newsletters, and by direct mail. I have commented on these tests earlier, but the issues are important enough to emphasize again.

Saliva hormone tests *only* measure the *free* hormone. The makers of the saliva test kits claim that a measurement of the free hormone in saliva gives a more reliable result than the combined fractions measured in serum. These claims have not been borne out in menopause research or fertility treatment settings.

Urine hormone assays are even less reliable than saliva. Urine tests measure only the metabolic break-down products of the various forms of the hormones, not the active forms. The urinary hormone tests are the most *indirect,* and least useful, measures of circulating levels of the active forms of the ovarian hormones.

Think about it, if you wanted to know how much money you had, would you *only* check what's in your pocket? Or would you want to know the amount in your pocket PLUS the amount in your checking account *and* the amount in your savings account? It seems only common sense that you want to know all three, and have a complete picture of your assets. The same is true for your testosterone "account."

If you just measure the free testosterone (or any other hormone) in the *saliva,* you miss having the crucial additional information provided by the *serum* test: the *free* portion that is available to immediately activate all receptors, the *weakly bound* portion available for activating certain receptors, and the *total* amount held in reserve by SHBG to be released and used as needed.

I tried saliva tests for patients and was greatly disap-

FACT:

If you don't know all three forms in your blood "testosterone account," it is difficult to determine the correct hormone dose or avoid unwanted side effects.

pointed in the extreme variation and lack of accuracy. I stopped using saliva hormone tests over a *decade* ago because of these problems. In women in whom I tested both serum and saliva at the same time of day, the two results were so far apart that it was like looking at two different people. The saliva values were all over the map, and never correlated at all with what the women themselves were telling me about their symptoms.

It is a major concern to me that women are making important hormone decisions based on only the saliva test of a few free hormones, often done in their local pharmacy without any other medical test results to give a complete picture of health issues and needs. Based on reputable medical studies, saliva tests cannot properly decide what treatment you need with something as critical to your health and as complex as hormones.

Serum tests, on the other hand, correlate **very** well with what my patients were telling me about how they felt. I feel strongly that such tests should be available to women, especially those who have had their ovaries removed.

Current international research has confirmed what I found in my own practice. Studies have compared the saliva and serum results in the same person, at the same time of day, and also correlated these samples with other objective tests, such as endometrial biopsy to check actual hormone effects on the tissue. Researchers found that serum tests gave consistent results to identify the type of hormone deficit, but saliva tests vary so much as to be totally unreliable. Medical references on this issue are included in the bibliography in Appendix I.

If you are going to the expense and effort of having your hormone levels checked, I urge you to work with a knowledgeable physician to have the "gold standard" serum (blood) tests and give you the most complete picture possible of your hormonal balance. In my opinion, hormone blood tests are helpful, effective, and provide psychological benefit by identifying a physical cause of the disturbing symptoms women may experience at mid-life and around menopause. Properly done serum hormone tests are also, in my experience, very *cost-effective*. There are too many "hidden" medical, psychological and relationship costs if you don't know your physiological measures. You may find that it is too expensive **not** to have this information as you plan how to best achieve your health goals.

I continue to use the "gold standard" serum hormone tests that are used in worldwide hormone research. They are much more reliable and clinically useful to me as a physician to help women check for overlooked health risks and then design appropriate hormone therapy strategies.

What Other Tests Should Be Done?

When we consider the *hundreds* of functions that our hormones oversee throughout the brain and body, it's no wonder that *hormone health* and *balance* is critically important. Because it's so important to have this optimal balance for *your* individual needs, I have called my approach *Your Hormone Power Life Plan®*. I summarized at the end of this chapter the steps for you to take to put this into action.

Your Hormone Tests and What They Mean

Ovarian Hormones : Ideally, a baseline estradiol, progesterone, testosterone, DHEA, and DHEA-S should be done in your 20s or 30s when you are feeling really well. Having your healthy baseline gives you a target range to aim for with any later hormone replacement. Unfortunately, this is rarely done. These same tests are even more important as we get older and start having symptoms. If you are still menstruating, you need to check levels at the low point of the cycle (days 1-3)

FACT

A comprehensive medical evaluation with reliable tests of hormones gives you critical information to help design an integrated plan for long-term success.

and also check the ratio of estradiol to progesterone in the luteal phase (about day 19-22). If you have stopped menstruating, or have had a hysterectomy, checking all of the ovarian hormones once for your baseline will usually do. Recheck these levels as symptoms develop, or intensify, after a tubal ligation, after hysterectomy, or when you start or change your hormone Rx. Checking levels after starting hormone therapy helps you be certain that you are above the currently accepted thresholds for preserving bone, brain, heart and other benefits of estradiol.

Here is a brief summary of what I have found over the years to be optimal ranges for the ovarian hormones:

Estradiol: In my clinical experience, women typically experience their usual energy level, mood, sleep, and memory when serum (blood) levels of estradiol are *above* 90 -100 pg/ml, which is the lower end of the range for healthy menstrual cycle levels. Levels up to about 200 or so, are the normal estradiol levels reached in the first half of the menstrual cycle before women reach menopause. At ovulation, estradiol levels are typically in the range of 300-500 pg/ml, and then in the luteal phase of the cycle (when progesterone is produced), a healthy level of estradiol is generally in the range of 200-250 pg/ml.

For restoring hormone function and health benefits after menopause, estradiol levels below about 90 pg/ml are generally too low to provide adequate relief of symptoms from hot flashes to muscle –joint pain and disrupted sleep and memory, not to mention maintaining a normal feeling of well-being. International research has found that estradiol levels below about 80-90 pg/ml result in increased bone loss after menopause. Cardiovascular benefits of estradiol have been found to occur at levels above about 80 pg/ml as a starting point. Therefore, I suggest you look for a level of about 90-100 pg/ml or better and then correlate this with your symptoms.

Wisdom:

Men and women require *different* amounts of hormones.

We *are* different.

Testosterone: In my experience, women typically experience their optimal normal energy level and libido when serum (blood) levels of total testosterone are between 40 and 60 ng/dl (which is 400-600 pg/ml using the same units for estradiol), with the percent of free testosterone at about 1-2% of the total. Levels below 30 ng/dl (300 pg/ml) are generally too low to maintain your usual libido, intensity of orgasm, energy level, and bone mass. The majority of menopausal women I have evaluated, particularly those who have had surgical removal of the ovaries in their thirties and forties, have had testosterone levels of less than 10...with barely detectable amounts of free testosterone. No wonder they don't have any sexual desire and feel tired all the time! Such low testosterone levels are also a significant factor in fatigue and low energy. As I described in Chapter 6, I usually measure the total, free and weakly bound forms of testosterone circulating in the bloodstream.

Heads Up!

Urine and saliva tests do not give as complete a picture of the hormone reserve that is available for action in the body, and I *don't* recommend them.

Levels of DHEA are discussed in Chapter 7, if you want to go back and read this material again. DHEA varies a great deal by age, time of day, and to a lesser extent can also vary by menstrual cycle phase. Be sure that you have the blood serum tests done to give a picture of both total and free hormones. **Urine and saliva tests do not give as complete a picture of the hormone reserve that is available for action in the body, and I don't recommend them.**

SHBG (Sex-Hormone Binding Globulin). This is a carrier protein in the blood stream that binds the sex hormones, holding them in reserve to release as needed to activate hormone target cells throughout the body. Measuring this protein in the blood helps us determine whether a hormone imbalance has also affected the production of this protein, which in turn will determine the relative amount of estrogen and testosterone in the free, active fraction in your blood. Too much free testosterone and too little free estradiol, for example, can adversely affect your appetite as well as determine the areas on your body where fat is stored.

SHBG is often abnormal in menopausal women and women with androgen excess, and returns to desirable ranges with appropriate treatment of the underlying hormone imbalance.

FSH. The **Follicle** ("egg") **Stimulating Hormone** is produced by the pituitary gland in the brain. Its main function is to stimulate the ovary to "ready" new follicles each month, for release at ovulation. When the ovary stops making optimal estradiol (for whatever reason), the FSH <u>rises</u> as the brain tries to stimulate the ovary to keep up estrogen production.

<u>High</u> FSH levels (above 20 MIU/ml) indicate that estradiol levels are too low, even if you are on hormone therapy. *If your hormone therapy dose is right for you* (and your brain), FSH comes back down to the lower level seen prior to menopause (less than 20).

In my opinion, FSH is <u>not</u> the most sensitive marker of estradiol decline, so that's why I check both the FSH (brain) and ovary hormones (estradiol, testosterone, and progesterone).

Thyroid: I recommend the following tests be done for women: TSH, free T4, free T3 and antithyroglobulin and antimicrosomal (antiTPO) antibodies, since these are more sensitive indicators of subtle (subclinical) thyroid disorders that may be affecting multiple symptoms and may also cause decreased ovarian hormone production. Since different labs have different units and reference ranges for free T3 and free T4, I can't give you specific guidelines here for those target values.

On most laboratory scales, hypothyroidism is usually diagnosed when TSH is greater than about 5, although many physicians don't treat with thyroid medication until the TSH rises over 8. Waiting until TSH is above 5, in my view, is waiting too long, and allows symptoms to get worse unnecessarily. In my opinion, it is better to begin thyroid medication sooner, rather than waiting until TSH has gotten to an arbitrary number because women can experience many problems, such as fatigue,

Wisdom:

Hormones levels fluctuate during the day.

It's better to check levels in the morning.

memory loss, muscle aches, low libido, weight gain, menstrual irregularity, infertility, PMS, and depression even when TSH is "only" 4 or 5, especially if the thyroid antibodies are also significantly elevated.

I may decide to start treatment even if the TSH is only 3 to 4, particularly when free T3 or free T4 are lower than optimal and women are having symptoms of low thyroid. This fits with current studies that indicate women may not have normal fertility or optimal ovarian function if the TSH is much above 2. The earlier treatment is begun, the less likely you are to have other adverse effects of low thyroid such as hair loss, muscle pain, high blood pressure, elevated cholesterol and serious weight gain, and the easier it is to regain optimal health.

Heads Up!

Women are often told their thyroid is normal, without having the complete thyroid tests done.

Keep in mind that if someone tells you that your thyroid tests are "normal," you still may have a subtle thyroid dysfunction contributing to your problems.

Of course, what most people, and many physicians, don't realize is that: (1) A "normal range" on a laboratory report is just that: a range. You may need higher or lower levels to feel well and to function optimally. I have always taught that we have to consider lab results along with the symptoms described by the patient and make a clinical judgment on all these aspects. After all, we are treating people, not lab values. (2) It is also possible that one or more lab measures may still fall in the lab "normal" range and yet other, subtle measures may be abnormal. I feel this is when it is very important to listen to the woman, and her descriptions of what is wrong, with an open mind and with trust in what she says and knows about her body.

Cortisol: This is the "stress" hormone produced by the adrenal glands. I recommend the 8:00 AM cortisol as a first step. If this is abnormal, then additional tests such as 4PM cortisol, free cortisol, and cortisol binding globulin (CBG) and other less common ones can be done. Levels that are too high may indicate a stress response to physical factors like sleep loss, hormone imbalances, medication side effects, drug use, and also to situational life "stresses." High total cortisol levels, but with normal free cortisol and high CBG, may occur in women taking birth control pills or oral menopausal hormone therapy as a result of the oral hormones causing the liver to make more of the binding protein, CBG. This isn't a medically serious problem, but there are other situations in which high cortisol can mean you have a different problem that may need treatment. Cortisol levels much greater than 25 µg/dl, when associated with high levels of *free* cortisol, could be a sign of Cushing's Syndrome. Extremely low morning cortisol levels (less than 7 µg/dl range) may indicate chronic stress effects (sometimes called adrenal "exhaustion" or adrenal insufficiency), or the more serious Addison's disease (*Adrenal Insufficiency*, or *AI*). If your cortisol is out of the desired healthy range, there are additional tests that can be done to decide the cause and appropriate treatment.

Prolactin: This hormone is produced by the pituitary and can be measured in a simple, reliable blood test that is best done between 7:00 to 8:00 AM in the morning. Elevated prolactin can be an indication of a pituitary hormone-producing tumor. These are usually benign, but may cause problems because (a) the tumor is large enough (macroadenoma) to cause pressure on the optic nerve resulting in visual changes, or (b) the hormone production from a small tumor (microadenoma) is enough to cause nipple discharge and disrupt ovarian cycles, which causes loss of menstrual periods, low libido, depressed mood, weight gain and other problems.

If the levels are too high, and there are visual changes, generally an MRI of the pituitary is done to see whether the best treatment is medication to bring down the prolactin, or whether surgical removal may be needed to prevent permanent damage to the optic nerve. Dopamine boosters (*agonists*), such as bromocriptine (Parlodel), cabergoline (Dostinex) and pergolide (Permax) are the most common medications used to treat elevated prolactin. High prolactin levels respond very well to these medications, so this problem is treatable— it doesn't need to continue to sabotage your health.

Your Bone Markers and Other Tests

N-telopeptide (collagen cross-linked NTx): This is a break-down product of bone that can be measured in blood or urine. If the urine test is used, it must be the *second* morning urine specimen to be accurate. If the body is breaking down bone faster than it is making new bone, NTx will be high (greater than 35). If you are "in balance" and the body is making new bone and breaking down old bone at about the same rates, this number will be low, or less than 35.

If the NTx is too high, even if your bone density is still good, it indicates that you are already beginning the process of excessive bone breakdown and are at higher risk for later life fractures. You should be taking more aggressive steps now to preserve bone, since just taking calcium and exercising regularly will usually not be enough to reverse this process. If you are taking hormone therapy to preserve bone, or taking medications such as Actonel, Fosamax, the goal is to have an NTx of about 35 or less.

CA 125: a cancer antigen that may be elevated in both ovarian cancer and several benign conditions such as fibroids, ovarian cysts, endometriosis, adenomyosis, and early pregnancy. I find this a useful component in evaluating women because it is a useful clue to the presence of *unrecognized* benign conditions that have to be addressed in planning appropriate treatment.

CA 125 is also currently the only available blood test that could alert us to an ovarian malignancy and is the best "early warning" test we have at this time, even though it is not diagnostic for ovarian cancer. I think it is important to have done if you have a family history of ovarian cancer, or if you have vague abdominal symptoms (gas, bloating, distension, change in bowel movements, pain, etc.) that are not responding to other measures.

Ferritin: This is a measure of the body's iron stores. Optimal levels for women are about 60-90 ng/ml. The concern about iron and heart disease is that *high* ferritin levels indicate excess iron that may increase your risk of heart disease. If your serum ferritin is in the normal range, it is fine to continue multivitamins that contain iron.

Low ferritin levels (generally less than about 40) are much more common in women due to menstrual blood loss over the years, and low ferritin is associated with restless legs, restless sleep, and symptoms of fatigue, muscle pain, poor exercise tolerance, hair loss and joint aches. If your levels are low (even without anemia yet showing on your hemoglobin and hematocrit), I suggest taking a multivitamin that contains iron. You may also want to discuss with your physician whether to add an additional iron supplement such as Slow-Fe or Niferex until ferritin is above 60.

High ferritin levels (i.e. over 150) are more common in men, and are not seen as often in women because women have monthly loss of iron in menstrual blood. High ferritin can indicate an iron storage disorder, and may cause damage to liver, kidneys and brain as well as cause a whole host of other problems such as fatigue, weakness, muscle and joint pain, diabetes, and in men, impotence. If ferritin is high, it is important to avoid taking multivitamins that contain iron, and consider donating blood at the Red Cross to decrease your iron stores.

Hemachromatosis is a hereditary disorder leading to iron overload. You should ask your physician about having further tests to determine whether you have hemochromatosis if a high ferritin is not related to taking iron supplements. You may request information from the American Hemochromatosis Society website.

Finding "Optimal" Levels verses "Normal" Reference Ranges

Getting your hormones and other labs checked can often be confusing when the results come in and your physician says everything is "normal" because the tests within the lab's "normal" range. This may be quite misleading. First of all, the reference ranges for women's ovarian hormones in particular are often too broad to be meaningful. Secondly, you have to consider that a given number is not necessarily the "optimal" number for you to feel best. If your estradiol or testosterone or thyroid is at the bottom of the normal range, that may not be enough to give your brain and body the "hormone power" fuel it needs for optimal performance. On the other hand, sometimes your hormone levels may be slightly higher that the "normal" range, but this may be where you feel the best. Ultimately, my medical approach is to listen to what you say about how you are feeling, and not just treat lab numbers. My desire is to carefully integrate the lab results with what you describe so *together* we can make the best decisions about appropriate treatment approaches for you.

Benefits of Comprehensive Hormone Testing

Other physicians have often been critical of the test recommendations I have just discussed, saying that it is "too expensive" to check women's hormones. I think it is too expensive *not to* know what is happening with these crucial metabolic regulators in your body. Besides, it is difficult to put a price tag on improving someone's quality of life. I think in the long run it is less expensive to check hormone blood levels than to do all the myriad tests and evaluations that I see women having done because hormone problems are not recognized. It also does not make sense to me (in time or economics) for women to undergo a series of psychotherapy sessions

Drugs Associated With Adverse Effects On Sexual Function

Antianxiety agents and Sedatives
- Barbiturates
- Benzodiazepines – examples: Valium (diazepam), Ativan (lorazepam), Xanax (alprazolam), Klonopin (lorazepam), and all others in this class
- Meprobamate (Equanil, Miltown, Meprospan, and others)

Anticonvulsants
- Carbamazepine (Tegretol)
- Ethosuximide (Zarontin)
- Gabapentin (Neurontin)
- Lamotrigine (Lamictal)
- Primidone (Mysoline)
- Trimethadione (Tridone)

Antidepressants
- Tricyclic antidepressants
- Monoamine oxidase inhibitors
- Selective Serotonin Reuptake Inhibitors
- Misc antidepressants (e.g. Remeron, Effexor)

Antihypertensives (Blood pressure medications)
- Calcium channel blockers
- ACE inhibitors
- Beta blockers
- Clonidine (Catapres)
- Methyldopa (Aldomet)
- Prazosin HCl (Minipress)
- Reserpine
- Spironolactone (Aldactone)
- Thiazide diuretics

Antipsychotics
- Seroquel, Zyprexa, Rispendal, Clozapine, Loxitane, Moban
- Butyrophenones (Haldol)
- Phenothiazines (Thorazine, Mellaril, Compazine and others)
- Thioxanthenes (Navane, others)

Miscellaneous
- Alcohol
- Anticholinergic drugs
- Chemotherapeutic medicines
- Cimetidine (Tagament)
- Clofibrate (Atromid-S)
- Digoxin (Lanoxin)
- Glaucoma medications
- Marijuana
- Metoclopramide HCl (Reglan)
- Narcotics
- Nicotine

> This table was prepared from multiple sources, such as the PDR, medical publications, and clinical work I have done over my entire career assessing these issues.

thinking that their problem is just due to stress or empty nest or a bad relationship.

Clearly, having reliable information about hormone levels has made an enormous difference to the women who had been told their symptoms were "all in their head" and who now have a hormone regimen that is right for them. Many of my patients have been able to stop expensive medications to lower blood pressure and cholesterol, as well as eliminate a variety of pain or antidepressant or sleeping medications when their estradiol levels were again in the optimal ranges.

In my opinion, the hormone blood tests are efficient, reliable, cost-effective, and psychologically helpful in identifying a physical cause of excess weight gain at mid-life and around menopause. There are too many "hidden" medical, psychological and relationship costs if you don't know your physiological measures. You may find that it is too costly to your quality of life **not** to have this information as you plan how to best achieve your health goals.

Beyond the Blood Tests: Putting It All Together

Hormonal imbalance is commonly not recognized or is misdiagnosed, so it is important for you to seek a thorough evaluation in addition to the hormone assays. There are many other, often incorrect, diagnoses given to women who, in fact, have declining estradiol, insulin resistance, PCOS, PMS, or menopause: some of these are mental disorder, manic-depressive illness, major depressive disorder, atypical depression, chronic fatigue, chronic candidiasis, panic disorder, anxiety disorder, stress reaction, and others. The goal of a comprehensive evaluation is also to make certain that you do not have another medical problem causing similar symptoms; and to insure that any previously unrecognized secondary disorders, which may be contributing to your symptoms, are diagnosed and properly treated.

Once you have the results of your various tests, You and your physician should then review this information together, and explore in the next chapter ways to boost your hormone levels to the optimal ranges I have described to help you restore a healthy metabolic balance so that all the other strategies will work more effectively. If you are having difficulty getting your hormone concerns to be taken seriously, however, it may be helpful to locate a specialty clinic to focus on these issues and give you more helpful resources and suggestions.

I have designed the *HER Place*® programs in Tucson and Dallas-Ft. Worth, Texas to help women get hormone levels properly tested, and to identify hormonal and other factors contributing to sexual problems, loss of energy and mood changes that can occur at midlife.

We feel that a comprehensive evaluation of all these factors is important to get you started on the right track, with objective information that guides you in making the right choices to improve your health. For those of you that are not able to visit us for a consult at *HER Place*®, these are the recommendations that I think are important for you to pursue in your local health care settings to provide the best possibility of identifying the factors that may be interfering with your progress.

The brands of transdermal estrogen patches along with Estrasorb lotion and Estrogel are recent innovations. Their delivery of the human 17-beta estradiol is the most "natural" of all. The estradiol is absorbed through the skin, directly into the bloodstream, much like the ovary does before menopause, without going through the stomach and liver *first*.

The estradiol patches all look like a clear circular, oval or rectangular "Band-Aid" that sticks to the skin and stays in place for several days as the hormones are slowly absorbed. As the hormone delivery falls, the patch is replaced. Each brand of patch lasts for a slightly different time, and because women metabolize the hormones at different rates, it can take some experimentation to find the right change schedule and dose strength for you.

Transdermal patches are a very good option for estrogen therapy, with only two primary drawbacks: (1) the skin irritation from the adhesive bothers some women, and (2) if you have a low level of HDL, you may need the extra "plus" of oral estrogen stimulating the liver to make more HDL. The patches (as well as Estragel and Estrasorb) gives the beneficial *physiological* (normal) effect of estrogen to maintain the normal level of HDL cholesterol, but not the *pharmacologic* (greater than normal) effect of extra liver stimulation to make more HDL as seen with the oral estrogens. If you have a normal cholesterol profile, the patch or estradiol lotion is all you need to give the physiologic benefits. If you have *high* total cholesterol and *low* HDL, an *oral* form of estradiol provides greater *decrease* in total cholesterol and *increase* in HDL for cardiovascular protective effects.

Effects of progesterone/ progestins on testosterone

Progesterone:

I use compounded natural progesterone for my patients, and we now have FDA-approved products available with Prometrium and Prochieve (formerly Crinone). For many women, the natural hormone progesterone causes fewer side effects than the synthetic progestins (Provera, Cycrin, MPA, norethindrone, levonorgestrel, etc), but there are also times when the potency of the synthetics provides better control of medical problems such as heavy bleeding or endometriosis. Some women just feel better on one of the synthetics than they do with natural progesterone. There is a great deal of individual variation, so don't get locked into the idea that one is *always* better than another.

Current accepted doses for progesterone to provide therapeutic effects on the uterine lining (endometrium) without excess buildup (hyperplasia) are as follows :

- For a **cyclic regimen,** the usual dose is 200 mg of **oral** micronized progesterone (i.e. Prometrium) for 10-14 days a month. If you are allergic to peanut oil you can't use Prometrium, but compounded prescription are available. **Prochieve** is a vaginal gel in sustained release form, and the 4% strength is given **every other night for 6 doses a month.** The FDA approved dose schedule gives 40 mg every other day, or an *average daily* dose 20 mg. If Prochieve isn't readily available, a similar preparation can be made up by a compounding pharmacist.

- For a **continuous daily regimen** the accepted dose is 100 mg *oral* progesterone every day, usually best given at bedtime because of the sedative side effects for most people.

- Note: *progestins* are more potent than natural progesterone, and are therefore used in much lower doses. For example, Provera or Aygestin 2.5 mg is usually given for a daily schedule, or 5 mg is used for 10-14 days in a cyclic regimen.

Please pay attention to this caution with progesterone! You can save yourself a lot of problems. There are many people recommending progesterone creams in doses of 100-200 mg per gram to be used daily. Research has clearly shown that progesterone doses in excess of 300 mg a day orally (or creams containing more than 20-30 mg per day) cause blood levels of progesterone that are as high as those found in the *third trimester of pregnancy*.

I see women getting prescriptions for 100 mg per gram of progesterone creams, to be applied twice daily. Such a dose is seriously excessive, particularly since the FDA-approved dosing for transdermal vs. oral is usually for transdermal forms to be about 1/10 a typical oral dose.

If you do the math, you can quickly see that 100 mg/gm cream is roughly equivalent to about 1000 mg oral progesterone. Two applications of such a cream each day

Wisdom:

Hormone levels fluctuate during the day.

Sometimes, it is better to divide the dose.

would give you roughly the equivalent of taking 2000 mg in a pill or tablet! No wonder women using this feel fat, bloated, fuzzy-brained, and depressed!

Higher doses of progesterone are often recommended for PMS treatment, but can cause or aggravate many other problems: (1) marked weight gain similar to pregnancy, (2) high blood glucose and decreased glucose control in diabetics or women with insulin resistance, (3) high triglycerides, (4) high cholesterol, (5) higher than normal insulin production, (6) more backaches, due to ligaments becoming lax or "loose" from progesterone effects, (7) headaches, or intensified migraines, (8) decreased sex drive, fuzzy thinking, decreased concentration, and (9) depressed, lethargic mood.

One problem is that many practitioners who recommend such high doses of natural progesterone do not check serum levels of progesterone, do not monitor the cholesterol-triglyceride profile, and do not check for changes in fasting glucose and insulin. They then miss these developing problems. In addition, excess progesterone often causes lethargy and fatigue. Be careful about too much progesterone, especially if you are overweight, have diabetes, hypertension, elevated cholesterol or triglycerides, or a history of depression.

If you think progesterone is a "wonder" hormone and doubt the potential for serious side effects with it, simply recall two common pregnancy-related problems most women know about: (1) pregnancy-induced ("gestational") diabetes, and (2) toxemia or pre-eclampsia, a severe form of high blood pressure that occurs in the latter part of pregnancy. These two problems often occur in the last stages of pregnancy when progesterone levels are at the highest levels.

If you use natural progesterone for hormone therapy, stick with the FDA-approved and medically-accepted dose ranges.

If you have difficulty tolerating progestins in other forms, a low dose option is Mirena, an *intrauterine* progestin-

Wisdom:

Your "hormone recipe" will be slightly different from your friends. The key is finding what is best for you.

delivery system approved as a contraceptive rather than as progestin therapy in peri- or menopausal women, but this is an option if you have side effects or continued low sex drive with oral progestins or natural progesterone. It releases only a very small amount of progestin daily directly into the lining of the uterus, and so there is very little progestin absorbed into the total body circulation to cause problems.

The low dose of progestin in Mirena, coupled with the higher delivery to the uterus, reduces the likelihood of the unpleasant side effects such as headaches, depression, low libido, weight gain, and vaginal dryness often associated with progestins in hormone therapy and birth control pills. Some perimenopausal and menopausal women use these intrauterine delivery systems successfully if they cannot tolerate any other form of progestin. A number of studies show that these products deliver enough progestin to effectively suppress the build-up of the uterine lining, and reduce bleeding problems.

Caution:

Combination drugs may seem convenient, but *usually* cause more problems because they are not *your* balance.

After a year, about 20% of women have no further bleeding, and this is a significant benefit in perimenopausal women who tend to have problems with erratic and heavy bleeding before menopause actually occurs.

There are some drawbacks, however, so it is important to discuss these with your health professional. Possible problems with Mirena include increase in ovarian cysts, increased risk of pelvic inflammatory disease if there are multiple sexual partners, increased risk of ectopic pregnancy, erratic bleeding, and menstrual changes. If you need a progestin and nothing else has worked, ask your doctor about these products. Pregnancy rates are less than 0.02%, and it also reduces the amount of monthly bleeding for most women after the initial 3-6 month adjustment. Synthetic progestogens (called progestins) are commonly used in birth control pills and HRT to regulate menstrual bleeding. Examples are medroxyprogesterone acetate (Provera, Cycrin), norethindrone (Aygestin, Micronor), norethisterone, norgestrel, levonorgestrel (in Mirena and many birth control pills), drospirenone (in Yasmin), etonongestrel (in Nuvaring), and others. Many women may actually feel better on some of these than on natural progesterone. It is important to keep an open mind and be willing to try different options.

In Summary

There is a systematic way to work with a variety of hormone approaches to correct health problems, relieve troublesome symptoms, and achieve your goals. There are many, many options to try. If at first you have problems, don't give up. Work with a knowledgeable health professional to create a hormone supplement program fine-tuned to your body needs that restores balance to your natural levels. It can be done.

Don't expect quick solutions to complex problems, however. It takes time, persistence and patience. If you have complex problems and many different symptoms, or are sensitive to medications, it could take six to twelve months to find exactly the right combination for your needs so your body can heal and repair for overall improvement. There are reliable, objective measures that will help you track your progress, in addition to your observations and feelings. Don't settle for feeling lousy every day. Don't continue what doesn't work. There are a variety of ways to rekindle your sexual spark, energy level, and vitality.

Your Hormone Power Life Plan®
Dr. Vliet's STARTING STEPS:

1. Examine your own health risks: Look for symptom patterns, diagnosed diseases e.g. high cholesterol, high blood pressure, diabetes, osteoporosis, and others.

2. Check your family history: Look for first-degree relatives (parents, siblings) with common problems that may affect your health risks, such as diabetes, PCOS, elevated cholesterol, heart disease, high blood pressure, thyroid or adrenal disorders, hypoglycemia, history of obesity. Check for other hereditary problems such as autoimmune disorders, depression, osteoporosis, dementias, or cancers that play a role in your own risks, and provide clues to how important it may be for you to have optimal hormone balance as you get older.

3. Work with a physician who will do objective tests: Look for one who uses standardized laboratory procedures and blood (serum) measures. To start out, I recommend the following (described in more detail later in the chapter):

(a) *Serum levels of all of your ovary hormones.* At a minimum, you need FSH, estradiol, progesterone, testosterone, DHEA, and DHEA-S

(b) *Serum cortisol, TSH, free T3, free T4, thyroid antibodies*

(c) *Fasting lipid profile* (cholesterol, HDL, LDL, triglycerides)

(d) *Metabolic profile* to check electrolytes, liver function, calcium, etc.

(e) *Fasting glucose and insulin, plus HgbA1C (glycosylated hemoglobin)* and a *2-hour post prandial glucose and insulin* (if waist is more than 30 inches).

(f) *C-reactive protein, homocysteine* to have a baseline check of potential risk markers for cardiovascular disease.

(g) *Bone density of the hip and spine.* DEXA is the most reliable test) to measure your "bone bank account." If you are under age 65, do not rely on heel and wrist/forearm tests of bone density, since in younger women these tests are not well-correlated with how much bone you have at the hip and spine. It's the hip and spine sites where fractures are more common and more debilitating as women get older.

Your Hormone Power Life Plan®
Dr. Vliet's STARTING STEPS:

(h) *Urine or serum test of N-telopeptide,* a measure of the rate of bone building vs. bone breakdown. Numbers greater than 35 mean you are breaking down bone faster than you are building it. This test is also useful to monitor your response to any therapy you may start, such as hormones or medications like Actonel or Fosamax.

4. Evaluate your lifestyle: Eliminate the hidden thieves of your sexual vitality. Limit use of alcohol; stop smoking tobacco. Don't use marijuana. Exercise daily. Balance your diet with the right mix of protein, fat and complex carbs. Worjk with your health professionals to reduce or eliminate medications that block you sex drive. Make sure you get your vitamins and minerals. Check out the OTC herbs or supplements—many can adversely affect your ovarian hormone balance, especially in premenopausal women. Make a list of the things you are doing *right*, and give yourself a gold star. Make a list of the unhealthy habits you want to change, and BEGIN NOW to change them.

5. Take stock of your stressors. Make a list of the ones you can change and *want* to change, as well as the ones you can't change right now. Begin thinking about ways to relieve excess stress in your life.

6. Take stock of your relationship, and work to rekindle the spark! Women's interest in sex is affected greatly by the quality of their relationship. If you and your partner are having problems with communication, or feeling like you are two ships passing in the night because your interests have diverged, consider couples therapy to help you get back on track.

7. Improve your love-making techniques. Many times couples don't realize that we can all learn new techniques for sexual pleasuring. There are many good resources to help if you feel bored or burned out with all the same old approaches you've used for years.

©Elizabeth Lee Vliet, MD 1995-2005

Chapter 10

Become the Savvy, New You! Putting it All Together

As you now know, testosterone and other hormones play crucial roles in maintaining a healthy sex drive and response. Hormones alone, however, are not the only element.

The *quality of the relationship* plays an even more critical role in sexual arousal for women. Male sexual response is more purely "biologic" than women's. Female sexual desire clearly has biological components stimulated by optimal estradiol and testosterone. For women to become fully sexually aroused, it is equally or even more important to have satisfying emotional-intimacy connections.

Do a "relationship check"

Ennui in the relationships, boredom with sexual technique, undue performance expectations—all can lead to loss of interest in sex for either/or both of you.

If there are problems and conflicts, work with your partner and perhaps a therapist to resolve those conflicts, improve communication and restore those positive feelings. Take time for sensual encounters to enhance intimacy and this will help re-ignite those sexual desires that may seem to be waning as you get older.

Jazz it up

Add some variety and spice to your sexual times. Try something new. Try a new place. Be spontaneous. And focus on appreciating each other. Taking each other for granted adversely affects your sexual responsiveness.

FACT:

For women to become fully sexually aroused, it is equally or even more important to have satisfying emotional-intimacy connections.

The most important words in marriage vows may be "to cherish." Show that you cherish each other with little daily kindnesses, caring gestures and words. All of these help foster feelings of being cherished by our mate, making the bonds grow stronger, love grow deeper. Without them, sex and the relationship suffer. Focus on showing your love throughout each day, not just during sex.

Wisdom:

You love
your
partner?

So..
TELL your
partner!

The idea that love and romance belongs only to the young is simply wrong. Studies have found that 70% of couples aged 60 to 93 enjoyed happy sexual experiences into their 70's, and some into their late 80's. Ill health is often the main reason that couples "give up" on sex. Others just "drift apart," and feel like sex is over.

Don't let that happen. Talk about what you'd like to change or improve. Seek professional help to check for medical problems that can be improved. Read books, see a counselor. Try the Sensate Focus experience, described below. Make time for each other. Work to rekindle the spark. It's worth the effort.

Spicing things up and trying new tools and techniques may be the answer to feeling that sex is monotonous in a relationship. Vibrators are one option that can help a woman learn to have orgasms by giving steady, rhythmic stimulation that leads to orgasm and teaches her what that sensation feels like. Vibrators should be seen as a helpful extension of the sexual experience, not just a sex toy. They can help a woman learn to 'let go,' which is necessary for orgasm. You can use a vibrator in as many different ways as you'd use manual stimulation. You and your partner can use it together to enhance stimulation for both of you.

Experts recommend a vibrator that is designed for massaging—one with a handle and a small round head to be used to stimulate the clitoris rather than the large, penis shaped ones designed to be placed inside the vagina. Embarassed at the thought of owning a vibrator? Try the jet of a spa tub. The vibrations can be intense like a vibrator and can help you learn the sensations of orgasm in the privacy and comfort of your own bathroom.

Enhancing pleasure and trying something new helps us break out of a rut. You can try new locations or positions. Add a touch of luxury to the bedroom or get away for a luxurious weekend. Change your normal routine to stimulate interest and end the monotony. Use the many books and resources I list in the Appendix to give you ideas and serve as your guide.

Sensate Focus

This is a series of sexual pleasuring exercises is designed to help you explore each other's bodies and communicate your feelings to each other so as to help each of you learn what is most pleasing, arousing, and desirable for the other. It is especially helpful to use when women have experienced pain during intercourse, yet want to overcome fear of penetration and still enjoy a sexual encounter. You may also do this alone if you do not have or want a partner. This series of exercises is described in more detail in the table that follows, or you may read more in some of the books I have included on the resource list.

Briefly, the Sensate Focus Experience establishes a structure to help both of you relax and not feel pressured to perform sexually and always proceed to intercourse. Prior to reaching Level IV, couples agree to abide by the guideline of no intercourse, no matter how sexually aroused you become. Keeping this agreement helps build trust and reduce performance anxiety. You and your partner commit to a specified amount of time, for example an hour or more. Select a time and place when you won't be interrupted and are able to "tune out" stressful stimuli. You may want to help create the desired mood with music, candles, pleasant fragrances, and sensuous fabrics.

One person begins as the receiver of the sensate pleasuring, and the other person is the giver. In the next time together, you alternate roles. During the

Don't stint:

Foreplay AND afterplay make for better sex.

Be inventive.

Make sex last.

entire time of the session, the giver caresses, touches, and explores the receiver's body. The receiver gives positive feedback about what feels pleasurable, what is less desirable and what is uncomfortable.

What does one do during these pleasuring times? Be creative! You may also have to redo the "mental tapes" from childhood prohibiting touching various body areas. Nothing is off limits for you as an adult unless it causes discomfort or pain for the partner. You may find ideas in some of the resource books in Appendix II. If you commit to this process, and communicate with each other positively and sensitively, you will likely find the "fires" rekindled in your sexual encounters.

Focus on Sensual Pleasuring

In a private softly lit comfortable place, usually the bedroom, undress and take turns touching each other's body, excluding breasts and genitals. You may touch, hold, kiss, lick, suck or otherwise caress your lover's body in a way that is pleasant and interesting for you as long as it doesn't cause pain or discomfort for the other person.

Your responsibility to each other is to communicate how you feel, expressing it positively rather than as a negative "Don't do that." You may communicate nonverbally by guiding your partner's hand over any part of your body or in any manner that suits you.

Some examples:
"Your rubbing makes me feel warm and secure."
"I like what you are doing now."
"Your kisses make me tingle."

If your spouse or lover caresses you in a manner that does not please you, you must take the responsibility for indicating this. However, instead of making a complaint, you might say, "It feels better when you press my lips more gently," or "I would enjoy a soft touch more."

You may want to try using lotion, oil, or even caressing with feathers or materials to explore the different sensations that are possible. Feel free to experiment.

While you are receiving, soak up every sensation, and enjoy the here-and-now experience. Try not to let your mind wander beyond what you are feeling. If it does, bring yourself back to the experience.

Remember, though, that whatever or however you feel is OK. The only requirement is to be aware of your feelings and sensations, and focus on intensifying your sensory awareness.

Either of you may start. You decide who goes first. But remember to take turns. By taking turns, you are able to concentrate on your own feelings, whether giving or receiving. The sensual pleasuring time is for each of you to be focused on yourself. If you are touching each other simultaneously, it is more likely that you get lost in focusing on pleasing the other person rather than learning what arouses you.

Pleasing your mate is an important part of a sensual encounter, but too often, women especially forget to take care of seeing that they receive pleasure from the encounter. You are equally important. Concentrate on taking responsibility for yourself and your feelings.

Remember to plan ahead, allow yourself at least 1½ hours for each session, and plan to be together at least twice the first week so each of you has a time for your own sensual focus.

To Summarize
Sensate Focus Progression

I encourage couples to proceed, at your own pace, through the following levels of pleasuring each other.

Level I: non-erotic, non-genital pleasuring
Level II: erotic, non-genital pleasuring
Level III: erotic and genital pleasuring
Level IV: pleasuring that proceeds to intercourse

Lifestyle Thieves of Sexual Vitality

Thieves of sexual vitality bound in our lifestyles

Cigarette smoking (and other tobacco use) is a big culprit robbing you of sexual vitality and performance. Nicotine in all forms of tobacco products constricts blood vessels and decreases blood flow to the pelvic organs in men and women, which causes impaired sexual arousal and difficulty reaching orgasm.

In women, chemicals in cigarettes are toxic to the ovary follicles, causing death of follicles and decreased production of estradiol and testosterone that you need for optimal sexual drive and responsiveness.

Nicotine affects men adversely by decreasing blood flow to the penis, which markedly reduces fullness and firmness of erections. As men get older and there has been cumulative vascular damage from use of nicotine, the problem gets worse.

Alcohol is another thief of sexual vigor. Alcohol is a depressant drug that dampens down the brain centers for arousal and orgasm. If you drink alcohol daily, it decreases your sexual desire and your ability to respond to sexual stimulation. It has a numbing effect on nerve endings. A small amount of alcohol may initially re- lease your inhibitions and make you feel relaxed and "in the mood for sex." After that, the depressant effect of alcohol makes it harder to reach full arousal and orgasm. Men who have had too much alcohol often have difficulty achieving an erection that is full and rigid enough to allow satisfying intercourse. Alcohol also increases liver production of estrone and SHBG, which in turn lowers free testosterone in both men and women. No wonder it can have such negative effects on your sexuality!

Stress saps sex drive. A hectic lifestyle, and burning the candle at both ends, is another frequently over-

---

Fact:

Alcohol, stress, smoking, SSRIs, all zap sex drive!

looked thief of sexual interest and responsiveness. You may be simply too exhausted to relax and become aroused. Remember, the "flight or fight" adrenaline response evolved to help us escape danger, not to *relax and feel romantic*. If stress has your adrenaline system working overtime to keep up with the demands in your life, your sexual energy thoughts and energy are shoved to the back burner. Take time out to get away, slow down, relax, and enjoy the physical pleasures of relaxed foreplay and sexual exploration. Notice I said *take* time, not find time. Daily pressures constantly eat up our minutes. Given the busy lives we all lead today you have to establish your priorities and take the time for what is important to you—it doesn't just happen.

Medications are another thief of sexual vitality and interest. Medicines such as serotonin-boosting antide- pressants, mood stabilizers, beta blockers, blood pres- sure medication, diuretics, high progestin birth control pills, high dose progesterone creams, anti-anxiety and sleeping medications –all can blunt sexual desire. Many of these also cause difficulty having an orgasm.

Medical problems like Diabetes, vascular disease, hypo- thyroidism and other unrecognized medical disorders also cause of loss of sexual desire and problems with orgasm. If you have noticed a significant loss of sexual desire, or have painful intercourse, vaginal dryness, burning or itching, or have noticed it is harder to have an orgasm, it really is important to have a thorough medical checkup, and appropriate laboratory tests.

This checkup should include a physical examination by your primary care physician or specialist, laboratory tests of general blood chemistries, blood glucose, liver function tests, tests for sexually transmitted diseases, and hormone blood tests (especially thyroid, estradiol, and testosterone). If your hormone levels are too low, talk with your doctor about appropriate options, pref- erably with bioidentical hormones, to help you regain your sexual vitality, energy and wellbeing.

Fact:

Medical illnesses can sap sex drive and/or decrease orgasm

Get Going and Move That Body!

Exercise has a lot of well-publicized health benefits, but did you know it can also rev up your sexual energy? Recent studies show that exercise boosts levels of estradiol, testosterone and DHEA, and decreases cortisol. Exercise helps clear away sluggish feelings from stress overload. Plus, a fit body adds to your confidence, sense of self esteem, and helps you just feel sexier.

Wisdom:

Do your part.

Move that body!

Exercise helps renew your energy and heal damage from illness.

Before you start new exercise program, talk with your physician to identify any limitations or cautions. Once you have the green light from your doctor, figure out what you like to do, where you would like to do it, and what level you are now.

A comprehensive workout gives the most benefits. A good exercise routine should include a warm up, aerobic activity, strength training, flexibility, and cool down. A trainer or exercise physiologist can help you individualize a workout routine to meet your specific needs, determine an appropriate training heart rate, provide a little coaching motivation, and help you modify exercises to address any limitations as needed.

For most women who are not involved in a regular exercise program, I suggest starting with a basic walking program. Walking is easy, feels good, requires no special training or equipment, and gives you a sense of accomplishment, along with the energizing effects of more oxygen to your body and mind. Work up a light sweat but don't exercise until exhausted. Start with 15-20 minutes of brisk walking 3 days per week. Once you have established this routine, try to increase the duration about 10% per week until you are walking at least 30 minutes and up to 45-60 minutes to optimize aerobic benefits and fat-burning pathways.

If you find that just walking is no longer "enough" and you feel you need to increase the intensity of your routine, try adding light hand weights one-half or one-pound weights are fine, but don't overdo and add more than two pounds per hand. Find a route with more hills and/or try to increase your speed for short stretches at a time. To increase the intensity of your workout, use a treadmill to pace yourself. It helps keep you from slowing down too much when you get tired or bored! Or, you can try a stationary bike with the attachments that also uses your arms—this really boosts the cardiovascular intensity of your program.

Try a new exercise video or DVD at home to get you going. Consider joining an exercise class. This gives you a definite time commitment to exercise and means your exercise doesn't get set aside with distractions of your daily chores. There are many new types of classes available, from Pilates to Power Yoga. You can even try "sexual" or "exotic" dance classes for a fun change of pace from the standard aerobic dance classes of the past. Talk about a way to re-ignite the sexual fires... you may learn a few new moves to perform for that someone special!

In addition to improving your sexual energy, exercise helps build bone, increase lean body mass, reduce total body fat, increase metabolism, reduce risk for cardiovascular disease and certain cancers, as well as improve overall functioning of most body systems. Researchers also reported in the European Journal of Applied Physiology in 2003 that a single session of high impact exercise in early postmenopausal women boosted estradiol levels 20% two hours afterwards. Talk about a wonder medicine! You can't beat it.

It really doesn't matter as much **what** you do for exercise. What matters is that you are **doing** it. You will feel better mentally, physically, emotionally and sexually. You will feel proud that you accomplished a goal and more motivated to continue making positive lifestyle changes. You will also experience a boost in your self-confidence. There is nothing more sexy and attractive than a self confident woman who walks with a spring to her step and a sparkle in her eye!

Bored

Tired of your normal exercise rountine, try another?

Variety is a wonderful energy booster.

Healthy Eating For Energy and Vitality…*and Feeling Sexier*

Diet can play an important role in your ability to enjoy a healthy sex life. A good diet can support hormone production and function, enhance energy levels, help us feel confident in our body, and give us a body that we want to share with others.

Our fuel sources come from three main sources; Proteins, Fats, and Carbohydrates. Protein contains amino acids that serve as the basic building blocks for the body to grow, repair tissues, and fight disease. Proteins also provide fuel for energy. The conversion to glucose is slower with protein than with carbohydrates, so proteins in our meals help keep blood sugar levels steady for longer, approximately 2-4 hours as compared to 1-2 hours from carbohydrates.

I recommend that mid-life women consume 35% of their calories from protein at every meal and every snack. This means at least 1/3 of your calories should come from a protein source every time you eat. Note: If you are a vegetarian, you need to eat your vegetarian sources of protein in the right combinations so that you get all 28 of the essential amino acids. I have more on this in my book, *Women, Weight and Hormones.*

Fat also provides the body with energy. Fat is a highly concentrated source that provides 9 calories of energy per gram as compared to 4 calories per gram for protein or carbohydrate. Fat is even more slowly metabolized than protein, so it keeps blood sugar levels steady much longer, approximately 3-6 hours after you eat. The right balance of fat is crucial to help absorb fat-soluble vitamins and to provide cholesterol and essential fatty acids that are used to make a variety of hormones, including estrogen, progesterone, and testosterone produced by the ovaries. If you cut back on fat in your diet too much, your body doesn't have the building blocks it needs to make your ovarian hormones. A low fat diet can also lead to decreased libido and sexual response because of the decrease in these critical hormones to light the fire.

This doesn't mean that you don't have to watch the *types* of fat you eat or that you can eat all the fat you want. Limit your fat intake to 25-30% of your total caloric intake.

Remember that proteins contain fat, especially animal source proteins (including fish). Even though I recommend lean sources of protein, when you increase the amount of protein in your diet you will also be increasing the amount of fat in your diet. This doesn't leave much room for additional fats, spreads, sauces, gravies, etc.

"Trans" fats, such as the partially hydrogenated margarines and spreads popular today, are especially unhealthy. Trans fats increase risk of diabetes and heart disease. Reduce the amount of saturated animal fats and opt for the more servings of desirable *unsaturated* fats from vegetable sources.

The remainder of your calories should come from complex carbohydrate sources, roughly 35-40% of your daily calories. Carbohydrates are a good source of energy because they break down into glucose easily in the body. Sources include whole fruits, vegetables, and whole grains.

Try to avoid over-doing simple carbohydrates such as fruit juices, white breads, white rice, white potatoes, rice cakes or highly processed foods that break down rapidly and cause your blood sugar to spike. This triggers an insulin overshoot, followed by a "crash" in blood sugar that leaves you zapped of energy an hour or two later. Simple carb foods should be eaten in small amounts, preferably with some protein and fat sources to help prevent blood sugar swings.

The key to a healthy meal plan is a balance of complex carbohydrates, proteins and fats at each and every meal. For effective fat loss, your meal plan for each meal

Wisdom:

Capture the revitalizing power of all your body's hormones by sound nutrition.

and snack should be: 35% protein, 30% fat, and 35% carbohydrates. I call this Your Hormone Power Plan® and I have described it in detail in my book, *Women, Weight and Hormones*, along with sample meal plans and caloric guidelines.

You will have more energy throughout the day and avoid "sinking" feelings of low blood sugar between meals. This helps reduce cravings for sweets. Not only will you feel better because you have more energy throughout the day, you will sleep better and have more energy for more pleasurable recreational activities like exercise and sex!

Doctor, I Need To Talk!

Important:

Women's sexual concerns are no less important than men's.

Talking with your doctor about your sexual concerns may not be easy for either of you. Sexual health and sexual medicine has been slow in coming to traditional medical settings like your doctors office. Recognition of sexual dysfunction as a medical issue is increasing, so we are making gradual headway. It's a serious problem, affecting millions of people, so doctors need to be more proactive in addressing these concerns as part of a routine health evaluation.

A study conducted in the United States asked 2,900 men and women between the ages of eighteen and sixty years of age about the prevalence of sexual dysfunction. Approximately 24% of the women reported inability to achieve orgasm, 19% reported trouble lubricating, and 14% reported pain during sex. Hormone decline, as well as other triggers can cause all of these problems. With many new medical techniques and treatments becoming available, we need to be asssertive about discussing our concerns with physicians. Even if your doctor doesn't address these issues, he or she should not be uncomfortable if you open the discussion. If you sense discomfort or disinterest, ask for an appropriate referral.

Women's sexual concerns are no less important than men's. Look at all of the attention that has been given to erectile dysfunction, and the medications that have been developed and FDA-approved to help male sexual dysfunction. *It's time for women to be heard in healthcare settings too.*

Suggestions For Talking About Sexual Difficulties With Your Physician

1. Try to be open and honest. Make a list of key points ahead of the appointment to save time and keep your focus. Don't understate or overstate your problem(s).

2. Start by describing how you are feeling, and keep it simple. For example:

   ❧ "I don't seem interested in sex anymore,"

   ❧ "I have trouble reaching orgasm now. That's a change for me."

   ❧ "Sex has become painful. I don't seem to lubricate like I used to."

   ❧ "I'd like to discuss possible reasons for these changes."

3. Ask specific questions and give specific symptoms.

   ❧ "It hurts with penetration."

   ❧ "It hurts with thrusting."

   ❧ "I don't have much feeling in my clitoris now."

   Being too vague will only delay treatment, or make it harder for your doctor to understand, or worse, diminish being taken seriously with your concerns.

4. Ask what he/she thinks about your concerns. Ask if he/she has been able to treat other patients with similar concerns.

5. Your doctor's responses will be a good indicator if he/she is the right one to help you with this issue. If you sense discomfort, ask for a referral to someone who specializes in this field.

©Elizabeth Lee Vliet, MD 1987-2005

What To Look For in Seeking A Professional To Help with Sexual Dysfunction:

1. Look for someone who is empathic, non-judgmental, and willing to listen. Check credentials to see if this person has the appropriate training and experience to help you with your particular problem.

2. Look for someone who doesn't project his/her values or attitudes about sex onto you, the patient.

3. Ask about provisions for privacy with sensitive content. New HIPPA regulations mean that your medical records can be sent in their entirety to certain third parties (insurance carriers, other health professionals) *without your further consent.* **Ask if your discussions about sexual matters can be protected from further disclosure without your specific approval.** If you are worried about your discussions being subject to office gossip, ask how staff access to charts is regulated.

4. Make sure that your physician (or therapist) keeps the discussion focused on your needs and your specific questions, and maintains appropriate boundaries. Sexualized touching of patients during physical exams or during psychotherapy sessions is <u>never</u> appropriate. Most professional groups have ethical prohibitions against such conduct. If you have an experience that you feel is inappropriate, speak up to a responsible health professional.

5. Trust your "gut"—if you are not comfortable addressing these issues with the professional you are currently seeing, find someone you can talk with.

©Elizabeth Lee Vliet, MD 1987-2005

It's A New World Out There…Be Selective with Sexual Partners

Relationships often change at mid-life, and many women find themselves back in the dating arena after many years in a stable relationship. The "dating game" brings on many new challenges and concerns. As we talk about all the ways to invigorate your sexual life, I feel I would be remiss if I didn't address the issue of sexually transmitted diseases (STDs). Many women now in their forties, fifties, and sixties now dating again don't have the experience of having to watch out for the myriad STDs out there today. All of the STDs are far more common today than when many of you readers were becoming sexually active. Some, like syphilis, had almost disappeared only to have coming roaring back in recent years with the widespread increased number of people having multiple sexual partners and unprotected sex.

WARNING:

Don't take chances.

Some STDs can be life threatening.

Bacterial vaginitis, trichomonas, chlamydia, herpes (HSV), human papilloma virus (HPV or "venereal warts"), gonorrhea, syphilis and now AIDS. The list is daunting. While AIDS is the most feared STD, the others are far more common and may result in a variety of painful symptoms that rob you of sexual pleasure and vitality. And yet, women are still frequently too shy about asking male sexual partners to wear a condom for fear of hurting their feelings.

Why!?

Stop and think here.

YOU are important. Your health is your greatest wealth. Take care of it. You are the only one who can take steps to protect yourself. I will bluntly tell you that if a man is worth having you share your body to have sex with him, he should be concerned enough about your health to wear a condom. This is particularly true in new relationships, or even in long-standing relationships if there is any indication that your sexual partner has had sexual encounters outside of your relationship. With proper use of a latex condom, you markedly decrease your risk of getting STDs, unless you have unprotected oral sex with a partner who has an active infection.

For best protection against STDs, use of a high quality latex condom should be combined with use of a spermicidal foam or jelly. In recent studies, the most widely used spermicide, nonoxynol-9, has been shown to kill all of the bacteria and viruses listed above. If you are concerned about whether your partner will have a condom available, you can always carry your own supply and be in control of having one when you need it. There are even "female condoms" available now that you can insert yourself.

Warning:

For best protection against STDs, use of a high quality latex condom should be combined with use of a spermicidal foam or jelly.

The incidence of AIDS in women in this country has been largely underestimated until recently due to the fact that women in the early stages of the disease suffer different manifestations, such as chronic vaginal infections. This wasn't even initially included as one of the criteria symptoms of AIDS. Women with AIDS also frequently die of different causes and infectious illnesses than do men. The survival rate of women with AIDS is significantly lower than that of men, according to a study conducted by the Maryland Department of Health in Baltimore, in part because men with AIDS have been twice as likely as women to get AZT, a drug that clearly prolongs survival.

If the current trends continue, AIDS will be the fifth leading cause of death next year for women between the ages of 15 and 44. This is a major health risk. Failing to insist that that a new partner uses a condom could be potentially life threatening. Don't take chances. Be aware, and be prepared.

It's Called Quality of Life

Throughout this book I have talked about getting you back to where you are optimal. That level will be different for each woman. I firmly believe that each and every woman deserves to be considered and treated as an individual. It takes sometimes takes time to figure out what may be ailing each person, but when a good diagnosis can be made, and a mutually agreed upon treatment plan works, it is truly a rewarding event.

In all of my writings, and in my presentations, I feel it is important to stress quality of life as we head into the last half of our time here. I also recognize from listening to my patients that getting there is not always easy. I want to share with you two letters I received while writing this last chapter.

Dr. Vliet—

I want to write some of my story for your new book, so perhaps others will know that there is hope out there. I hope this is of some value to you. In my early forties, my menstrual cycles became alarmingly erratic. I was struck frequently by paralyzing headaches. Yeast infections became common. My body would ache. I really noticed my energy level decline. The headaches would be accompanied by nausea and would grow so intense that I was worthless at work or at home. My mood would swing violently into the dark zone. Retreat seemed to be my only option.

I had thyroid cancer when I was seven and my thyroid had been removed. Could my daily dose of Synthroid, taken to replace the gland's vital function, have something to do with this devastation? Was I prematurely menopausal? My mother had not experienced menopause until her early fifties. Was some other, possibly cancerous, predator loose in my body? Friends suggested anti-depressant medication, or even hinted that I was struggling to repress the effects of some powerful emotional trauma.

Consultations with gynecologists, both male and female, left me with a medicine chest full of topical ointments that barely suppressed symptoms, and a head full of the patronizing assessment that I was peri-menopausal. I was essentially told that this was

Fact:

You can't resolve problems until you more fully know the causes.

something that had to be endured, that I should be a big girl about it. At age 45 it was hard to adjust to the fact that feeling good might be a thing of the past, that these mysterious symptoms were going to be a fact of life.

One weekend, in the grip of all this pain, my husband and I went trawling in the women's health aisle of the bookstore. The bright cover of Dr. Elizabeth Vliet's book, Screaming To Be Heard, screamed at me from the shelf. I knew I needed to read this book. I inhaled it, experiencing the blessed relief that comes when one encounters writing that makes one feel sane and less alone. My experience was validated. Other women, including the author, had suffered similarly. Most importantly, there was something I could do about it.

Conventional Ob-Gyn's had offered me largely ineffective medications, and what seemed an antique assessment; that women's bodies are mysterious, and it was up to me to "tough out" this miserable season of my life. No one spoke to me about the body's ever-shifting hormonal balancing act. Dr. Vliet's book revealed that there were options other than resignation and despair. I needed to pay attention to my body, and I needed a doctor with both skill and compassion to pay attention with me.

I decided I wanted Dr. Vliet to be that doctor. I waited several months for my face-to-face appointment, filling out lengthy and probing questionnaires, and getting a panel of blood tests. Because she knows the information she will need, blood tests are done in advance so we could get right at the diagnosis and treatment plan. When I flew across the country to meet Dr. Vliet it never occurred to me that a consultation with a physician could be such a moving and exhilarating experience. During our two-hour consultation she told me many things, but she listened as well. She had clearly mastered all the anecdotal and clinical data I had sent her. She seemed to know me.

HEADS UP:

Don't let someone tell you such blood tests aren't available or are not helpful.

They are.

There is a rigor to Dr. Vliet's approach. She realizes that every woman's body chemistry is a unique phenomenon. The quick consultation and the gynecological cliche of "it's that time of life" are not for her. Whereas the unspoken message from many doctors I had turned to was "don't bother me," her plainly stated message was "tell me all you can" and keep telling me, over time. Every 4-6 months a comprehensive panel of blood work is ordered and then carefully considered along with my symptomatology. We discuss the options. My hormone regimen is carefully regulated. The close scrutiny of my blood chemistry is accompanied by subtle but forceful demands from Dr. Vliet to watch my diet, consider my vitamin intake, and to exercise. She also reminds me to take time for ME, and to make time in our busy life to be with my husband.

I feel so much better now. I feel like an adult who knows what is happening rather than a confused and victimized child. It took me a while to get used to this adulthood, to feeling worthy of such scrupulous care. I am not the true-believer or fanatical type but I do know that there are millions of women whose lives would be richly improved by this kind of experience. She has taught me to care for, and to care about, myself.

And the second letter from a long-standing patient talked about her quality of life as well, and the joy in regaining health:

As you know in 1996 I was diagnosed as hyperactive thyroid. After numerous consultations and efforts with my local physician I received nuclear iodine treatment, and was also put on a drug called PTU to regulate my hormones. I really felt the best I had felt in years. PTU is a drug you cannot continue to take because it is harmful to your liver with long-term use.

When the doctor started lowering the dosage I immediately started to feel differently. I became more depressed and difficult to be around, I did not have the energy I had before, I had less self-confidence, and I lost my libido. This was causing terrible anguish for me, and threatening our marriage. My husband thought I didn't love him any longer because I didn't have any desire for sex.

The physician informed my husband and me that I needed to see a psychiatrist; he could do no more for me. My husband suggested we leave and look for help elsewhere.

Not long after, one Saturday afternoon, I told my husband that I felt like screaming at everyone and everything. In desperation we went to a bookstore. In the women's health section my husband saw a book by Dr. Vliet titled "Screaming to be Heard."

He remembered what I had said, and quickly realized that the book outlined a number of my problems. He stayed up most of that night reading the book, highlighting all the things that seemed to apply to my situation. The one that stuck out so clearly was early in the book when Dr. Vliet said that if your doctor does not understand your problem, he will probably say you need a psychiatrist.

On Monday morning my husband was on the phone to Dr. Vliet's office. He wanted to know if she was strictly an author, or if she still saw patients, especially out of state patients. We scheduled an appointment halfway across the country from our home. Dr. Vliet reviewed my case and said, "I believe we can help you, but it will be a slow process because of the complexities of the thyroid situation."

We, as a couple, can honestly say that this book changed our lives. We had been married over thirty years and were desperately trying to hang on to our marriage and regain our sex life. There was some change almost immediately. But it took almost two and a half years of step-by-step adjustments to see the results we were all looking for. We are delighted *to say that the past five plus years have been the most happy and rewarding of our marriage.*

I am pleased with myself perhaps for the first time in my life. I have a positive attitude about almost everything, rarely feel depressed, my weight is stable, and I now have a great libido. Adding testosterone to my thyroid and estrogen made a huge difference for me. Life is good due to my husband's love of books, that led him to Dr. Vliet's book, and the road to a successful approach to regaining my joy of life."

To all of you readers: use the information in my books to give you a guide to working with *your* physician to improve your health. It is not about just being alive. It is about your quality of that life.

Self-Test: How's My Sexuality?
Introduction

I first wrote this questionnaire at the beginning of my career as a guide for my patients to use in helping them reflect on their sexual concerns in the privacy of their home, before their appointments with me or any other health professional. It has been clear that both men and women often feel embarrassed and awkward talking about sexual matters, and as a result, have a hard time initiating discussions about sexual problems with their physician.

This "Self-Check" was my attempt to try and make it easier for patients to think about their concerns, and then make a list of specific questions they wanted to discuss.

I hope you readers will also find it helpful. Take time by yourself to consider these questions, write down your responses.

There are no right and wrong answers to these questions. I have written them in hopes it will help you reflect honestly about areas you may wish to improve, or possible health issues that should be addressed with a professional you trust.

Self-Test: How's My Sexuality?

1. Am I satisfied with the frequency of my sexual activity? Has it declined in recent months or years? If so, what ideas do I have about causes? (Suggestions for reflection: think about your body, are you satisfied with how you look and feel?), your partner, your lifestyle (do you drink too much alcohol, use drugs or medications, smoke tobacco?), your stresses (are you overworked and too tired to relax and enjoy sex?), and others.

2. Am I as interested in sexual activity as I have been in the past? Is my partner healthy and interested in sex?

3. Do either my partner or I have any difficulty performing sexually?

4. Have I noticed a change or decline in my level of sexual desire?

5. Have these changes been sudden or gradual in onset?

6. Am I experiencing any pain or discomfort (burning, itching, bleeding, etc.) with sexual intercourse?

7. Have I been having decreased vaginal lubrication and feeling too "dry" to enjoy sexual activity?

8. Does it take longer or is it harder to achieve an orgasm, making me feel like it's just too much effort to try?

9. Am I experiencing painful muscle contractions (e.g. uterus) with intercourse or with orgasm, that inhibit my interest or desire?

10. Am I having any other body changes that suggest a hormone problem or other medical illness? If so, what are they?

11. Am I angry or upset with my partner and not communicating these feelings?

12. Have I felt a general loss of pleasure in my life, felt depressed, or had thoughts of hurting myself?

13. Are there other relationship problems (including my relationship with MYSELF) affecting my sexual activity and enjoyment?

14. What would I like to see changed or improved in my sexual activity and relationship with myself and others?

And in Conclusion...

Your sexual vitality and physical energy are integral and ongoing parts of your life. Neither one needs to screech to a halt at age 40 or 50 or 60 just because you are older. A significant part of our self-identity is feeling well, fit, and energetic as well as sexually attractive. We also want to feel well and healthy not only for ourselves, but also for those we love who are a part of our life. There is much you can do to achieve better health and zest.

Throughout this book I have focused on the role of hormones as your foundation for a healthy sex life, restored energy level, improved strength and vitality. Because testosterone is rarely thought of as a female hormone, and it is so important to our overall health, and more specifically our sexual health, I have made it the primary focus of this book. There are many other dimensions to consider too, of course, but in my practice experience, the most *overlooked* one is that optimal levels of testosterone and estradiol are essential for sexual desire and response.

And our overall health is governed in so many ways by our hormones. At our most basic level, we *are* our biology. The chemical soup bathing our brain and body needs its hormones to function optimally. Then our psychological and spiritual dimensions function at their best too. When your whole body—physical, emotional and spiritual—is in balance, it shows in your eyes, your walk, and your confidence.

Even though there are many possible causes of female sexual dysfunction, my view is that you must begin with an evaluation of the hormones that affect so many systems in our body including sexual function.

I have given you outlines of how to identify hormonally-triggered problems. I have listed symptoms that can give you clues to a hormone imbalance. I have explained the components of a comprehensive medical evaluation. There are reliable blood tests available to help sort out what you may need. There are optimal ranges to help you interpret the test results. Don't let someone tell you such tools aren't available or are not helpful. They are. I have discussed how you can also identify what's optimal for you.

I have described many different options for restoring hormone health. I want you to be empowered with the knowledge you need to get the most from your medical appointments, and to help you know when to seek help from therapists and other health professionals.

If, in a collaborative physician-patient relationship, we do things well and responsibly, you can restore energy, vitality...*and* your full sexual desire and expressiveness. To do that, let me repeat, we have to test, evaluate, prescribe, and test again to see if the medication and the method of delivery are appropriate. We then periodically re-test and re-evaluate, as our bodies change or adjust. When needed, consider therapy and other modalities to help address other aspects of your sexual response and relationships.

Live Longer, Live Fully

On average, women are now living another fifty years after our natural hormonal peak in our late twenties and early thirties for estradiol, testosterone and others. How do YOU want to live those additional years?

Make the most of your longevity.

Be a SAVVY woman. Take charge of your health, your sexuality, your energy, and act on all this information. Don't ignore it. YOU are worth it!

Going Forward!

- Be informed
- Be savvy
- Be strong
- Be sexy
- Be YOU!

Appendix — Glossary of Medical Terms and Abbreviations

Appendix I
Glossary of Medical Terms

This is a list of the medical abbreviations and a glossary of medical terms I have used throughout this book. If you are going to take charge of your health, it will help for you to become informed about what these terms mean, so you will understand terms used by your physician to explain what is happening to your body.

I. List of Medical Acronyms Used in This Book

Hormones:
E1 – estrone
E2 – estradiol
E3 – estriol
T4 – thyroxine (thyroid)
T3 – triiodothyronine (thyroid)
FSH – follicle stimulating hormone
LH – luteinizing hormone
SHBG – Sex Hormone Binding Globulin
TSH – Thyroid Stimulating Hormone
TBG –Thyroid Binding Globulin
GH – Growth Hormone

Measurements:
dl – deciliter
cc – cubic centimeter (1 cc=1 ml)
mcg – microgram
mg – milligram
ml – milliliter (1 ml = 1 cc)
ng – nanogram
pg – picogram

Other Terms:

BCP	birth control pill (see also "OC" for oral contraceptive)
BMI	body mass index
BMR	basal metabolic rate
BTL	Bilateral Tubal Ligation
CHOL	cholesterol
CVD	cardiovascular disease
CRP-hs	C-reactive protein, highly sensitive
DEXA	Dual Energy X-Ray absorptiometry
DA	dopamine
EPI	epinephrine
EFA	essential fatty acids
FFA	free fatty acids
GABA	Gamma Aminobutyric Acid
GLA	Gamma Linolenic Acid
HDL	high density lipoprotein ("good" cholesterol)

HRT	Hormone Replacement Therapy
HT	Hormone Therapy
IUD	Intra-Uterine Device
LDL	low density lipoprotein ("bad" cholesterol)
NE	norepinephrine
NTx	N-telopeptide (bone breakdown product)
OC, or OCP	oral contraceptive pill
PCOS	Polycystic Ovary Syndrome (also PCO)
PMS	Premenstrual Syndrome, also called PMDD – Premenstrual Dysphoric Disorder
SERMS	Selective Estrogen Receptor Modulators.
ST	serotonin, also called 5-HT (5-hydroxytryptophan)
TG	Triglycerides

II. Medical Terms Defined

Adrenal Glands: Two small glands situated on top of the kidneys, which secrete steroid hormones (cortisol, aldosterone, DHEA) and the stress hormones epinephrine and nor-epinephrine (sometimes grouped together in common usage and called adrenaline).

    Adrenal Insufficiency (Addison's)

    Adrenal Excess (Cushing's)

Affect (Affective): a term used to mean "mood" or range of emotional expression. "Affective" refers to emotional content or to disorders of mood.

AIS (Androgen Insufficiency Syndrome): Diminished production of androgens. Can occur in women and in men; more common with older age, and also has many caused in younger women (and men). FADS (female androgen deficiency syndrome) is term previously used. See discussions in text for causes and treatments.

Alopecia: Loss of hair that is excessive and abnormal. There are many medical, dietary, and lifestyle causes. Anorexia, bulimia and imbalances in estrogen, androgens, excess progesterone, and excess or deficiency of thyroid hormones are common causes in women.

Amenorrhea: The absence of menstrual bleeding in a woman who has not gone through menopause; may be due to prolonged stress, PCOS, thyroid disorders, excessive exercise, eating disorders, premature ovarian failure and others.

Amino Acids: Chemical molecules found in foods that serve as the "building blocks" for the body to make its proteins. Essential amino acids are those that the body cannot synthesize and that must be included in the food we eat. Dietary protein containing all of the essential amino acids is "complete protein" and can be obtained from animal/dairy products and also by combining any three of the following: nuts, grains, seeds, or legumes at one meal.

Anabolic: A term meaning "to build up," as in the anabolic phase of metabolism, a process of using nutrients to build larger molecules that are used by the body for growth, repair and healing. See also catabolic and metabolism.

Anabolic Steroids: Hormones that stimulate the growth of bone and muscle (lean body mass) and can have male ("virilizing") effects on body chemistry and shape if levels are too high for women.

Androgens: A group of hormones that produces masculine effects on the body. This group of hormones is produced by both the adrenal glands and the gonads (testes in males and ovaries in females). Androgens are produced in much smaller amounts in women compared to men. Androgens decrease with aging in both men and women, but after menopause in women the levels of androgens in women are higher relative to the amount of estrogen that remains. This change in balance of androgens to estrogen produces the characteristic body changes (waist area fat, hair growth on face and chin, etc.) seen in older women.

Androgenic: An adjective used to describe substances (natural or synthetic) that produce masculine changes in the body: stimulating male pattern hair growth (or loss), oily skin, acne, deepening of the voice, increased appetite, increased muscle mass, increased bone mass, and increased total cholesterol with lower HDL.

Androstenedione: An androgenic hormone produced by the ovaries, testes, and adrenal glands; excess levels in women (such as in PCOS) lead to unwanted facial hair, acne, infertility, body fat gain around the middle of the body, oily skin and other masculinizing effects.

Antibodies: Protein substances produced by the body (or transferred from a mother to infant during pregnancy) that react with foreign substances called antigens as part of our immune process. Antibodies are made to foreign tissue such as grafts, bacteria and viruses; antibodies may also be produced against our own body organs (thyroid, ovary, etc.) in the autoimmune disorders.

Antigen: A substance that triggers the formation of antibodies to stimulate an immune reaction; may be introduced from external sources (bacteria, viruses, etc.) or formed within the body.

Antioxidant: Substances such as vitamins A, C, and E, beta-carotene, and selenium, which protect the body's cells and tissues from oxidative damage caused by free radicals.

Atrophy: Wasting or thinning of tissues or organs.

Benign: Non-cancerous or nonmalignant.

Bioavailable: a substance, often carried in the bloodstream, that is unattached to carrier proteins and therefore able to bind to special receptor sites on cells throughout the body. The amount of a compound or hormone that is "bioavailable" is also called "active" or "free fraction."

Bio-identical: A molecule that is exactly the same make-up and configuration as those made by the body. Hormones that are "bio-identical" may be made in the laboratory from building blocks found in plants, but end up with the same chemical structure as the hormones made by body organs such as the thyroid and ovary. Bioidentical hormones are often called "natural" hormones, but "natural" may also refer to a biological source (such as the horse) that produces molecules different from those made by the human body. Bioidentical is a more correct term than "natural" when referring to the types made by the human body and pharmaceuticals that are designed to duplicate ones made by the body.

Bisphosphonates: a group of medications that prevent excess bone break-down, and stimulate the formation of healthy new bone. Examples are Fosamax, Actonel.

Body Mass Index (B.M.I.): A scientific way of determining body composition. It is calculated according to the formula B.M.I. = weight (kilogram)/height squared (meters). The normal B.M.I. for women ranges from 20 to 25 kg/m2 and many hormonal and menstrual problems can be overcome by keeping weight in the normal range.

Bone Resorption: the normal process of bone break-down or "remodeling" that occurs throughout our lives to allow healthy strong bone to replace older, brittle bone. Resorption can lead to osteoporosis if the bone building process slows down too much, and breakdown (or "withdrawal") of bone exceeds bone formation.

Bound Hormone: Hormone that is circulating in the bloodstream connected to a carrier protein (such as sex-hormone binding globulin, SHBG or corticosteroid binding globulin, CBG), and therefore is not "free" to be biologically active at cell receptor sites. (See "free hormone").

Breakthrough Bleeding (BTB): Irregular vaginal bleeding or spotting occurring in women when they are taking oral contraceptives or postmenopausal hormone therapy.

C Reactive Protein: A protein made by the liver in response to inflammation and also as a result of some medications being processed by the liver. A high level of C-reactive protein (CRP-hs) is a general marker in the bloodstream indicating the presence of inflammation of any kind, but it is also used as a marker of inflammation in blood vessels that could indicate the beginning of cardiovascular disease.

Calcium: a crucial mineral involved in maintaining normal bone strength/density, and normal nerve and muscle function.

Calcitonin (Thyrocalcitonin): a hormone produced in the thyroid gland that regulates calcium balance in the body

Cancer: A malignant growth/tumor with rapid multiplication of abnormal cells which may spread to and invade distant body parts.

Cardiovascular Disease (CVD): Disease of the heart, arteries, veins, and capillaries of the circulatory system, contributing to increased risk of heart attack, stroke, blood clots, and poor circulation in legs and feet.

Catabolic: A term meaning "to break down", as in the catabolic phase of metabolism, a process of breaking nutrients into smaller molecules that are either utilized by the body for growth and repair, or excreted through the skin, lungs, kidneys and bowels. See also anabolic and metabolism.

Cat Scan: A computerized X-ray of consecutive sections of the body, which is used to look for tumors, masses, and other abnormal structural changes inside the body.

Cell: The basic unit of structure of all animals and plants that carries out the physical functions of life processes, either by itself or working together with other cells making up organs.

Cellulite: Fatty deposits resulting in a dimply or lumpy appearance of the skin. It is gradually lost with proper fluid intake, exercise, and overall weight loss.

Cervix: The opening of the uterus that projects into the vagina. It is also called the mouth of the womb. Some women report that the penis thrusting against the cervix during intercourse leads to greater sexual stimulation and more intense orgasm, which may be a reason to leave the cervix if a woman needs to have the uterus removed.

Chlamydia: A sexually-transmitted bacteria that is a common cause of pelvic infection and infertility, may lead to premature ovarian decline or failure.

Chloasma: Brownish pigmentation of the face that can occur in pregnancy (may also be caused by some types of hormonal imbalance, and progestin-dominate birth control pills).

Cholesterol: An important body molecule that is the precursor for the body to make sex hormones, adrenal hormones, and other molecules. It is found in the blood in three forms: (1) High Density Lipo-protein (HDL), which protects against plaque formation in the arteries (atherosclerosis); (2) Low Density Lipo-protein (LDL), which promotes plaque formation (atherosclerosis); oxidized LDL is the form that damages the walls of blood vessels; and (3) Very Low Density Lipoprotein (VLDL), also a plaque promoter. Cholesterol is produced in the liver even when dietary intake is lowered, and it is found in all animal fats and oils (butter, milk, meat, cheese, etc).

Circadian Rhythm: the regular, rhythmic pattern of changes in biological activity and function that occurs over the course of a day. Examples of circadian rhythms are our sleep-wake cycle, the daily cyclic variation in cortisol and melatonin secretion, among many others.

Climacteric: The span of years in a woman's life when hormone levels are gradually decreasing, leading to changes in body shape and function ultimately ending in the last menstrual period. The climacteric represents the years of transition for women from full reproductive life to menopause.

Clotting Factors: substances carried in the bloodstream that promote coagulation (the process of clotting), such as prothrombin; thrombin; thromboplastin; calcium in ionic form; and fibrinogen. Clotting can be retarded by cold, smooth surfaces, and other substances. Clotting is hastened by warming or by providing a rough surface (such as plaque inside arteries). Medications may be given to promote or decrease clotting.

Clitoris: The female equivalent (embryologically) of the penis. It is a small bulb found at the top of the vulva, just below the pubic bone, and is covered by a hood of tissue. It contains erectile tissue and dense, highly sensitive nerve endings that are important in enhancing a woman's sexual arousal and orgasm. Clitoral nerve endings become less sensitive as women's ovarian hormone levels decline, whatever the cause, but especially at menopause.

Combined Oral Contraceptive Pill (OC): A contraceptive pill containing both female sex hormones, estrogen and progestin. (To contrast the combined OC, there are also progestin-only contraceptives (examples: Micronor tablets; Norplant and Depo-Provera are long-acting implants/injectables, and Mirena IUD).

Complex Carbohydrates: Carbohydrates are macronutrients that provide a quick energy source. Complex carbohydrates refers to those found occurring naturally "complexed" with fiber, minerals, and other nutrients (such as grains, whole fruits, vegetables). They are more slowly absorbed and utilized than processed or refined carbohydrates (sweets, pasta, white bread).

Conception: The fertilization of the female egg by the spermatozoa (sperm).

Conjugated Estrogens: A mixture of estrogens, chemically different from those made in the human female ovary, that may come from animals (Premarin®, horse), or plants (Cenestin®)

Corpus Luteum: The yellow-colored, progesterone-producing sac that is formed within the ovary from the remains of the follicle after it has released its egg at ovulation.

Corticosteroid: (also glucocorticoid) Any of a number of steroid hormones produced by the cortex of the adrenal gland. Cortisol is an example.

Cortisol: An adrenal cortical hormone (glucocorticoid), usually referred to as our body's "stress" hormone because it prepares the body to respond to emergencies or stresses. It is closely related to cortisone in physiological effects.

Cortisone: A steroid compound made naturally by the adrenal glands and also produced synthetically in laboratories for use as a drug. It has a powerful antiinflammatory effect, but may produce many adverse side effects with high levels over long periods of time.

Cushings Syndrome (Disease): A group of symptoms and signs such as moon-shaped face, buffalo hump, upper body obesity, and high blood pressure caused by excessive amounts of cortisone either produced by the body or taken as medication. Primary Cushing's Disease can be caused by adrenal or pituitary disease or tumors. Pseudo-Cushing's (also called Cushing's Syndrome) can occur in women with androgen excess, such as PCOS; it can also occur in people taking corticosteroid medications for other conditions, such as asthma or arthritis.

Cystic Acne: A skin disorder manifesting as blocked pores and pimples, many of which are blind cysts containing pus. It is a severe form of acne, often occurring in women with androgen excess, or women with excess progesterone relative to a low estradiol.

Daidzein: isoflavone compound (also called phytoestrogen) found in soy and other plants that has weak estrogenic effects.

DEXA: Dual Energy X-ray Absorptiometry, a highly reliable means of measuring bone mineral density using very small amounts of radiation. Recommended for women with multiple risk factors for osteopenia/osteoporosis, or women who want a baseline measure before beginning menopause. Measures of the hip and spine (rather than heel and forearm or wrist) are the most reliable measures in women under age 65.

DHEA: Dehydroepiandrosterone. One of the androgens ("male" hormones) produced in the adrenal glands and ovary in women. Excess levels cause facial hair, scalp hair loss, oily skin, acne, upper body weight gain among other changes.

Disogenin: A steroid compound found in wild yam and other plants that is used by pharmaceutical companies as a "building block" or precursor molecule to make bioidentical forms of human hormones such as progesterone and 17-beta estradiol. Disogenin in extracts of wild yam (found in skin creams) cannot be converted by the human body to progesterone, estradiol, DHEA or testosterone because we lack the necessary enzymes to do this.

Diuretic: A substance, whether synthetic or natural, that stimulates the kidneys to excrete salt (sodium chloride) and water, thereby relieving fluid retention. Some diuretics, such as HCTZ, act on the kidney and cause more loss of potassium as well as sodium. Other diuretics, such as spironolactone, help the body save potassium because they act on aldosterone, the body's fluid-regulating hormone.

Diurnal: Variation by time of day. For example, hormones in the body often are higher at one time of day and lower at another in a predictable pattern. Diseases may alter the normal diurnal pattern. An example: melatonin is normally highest at night (promotes sleep) and lowest in the bright sunlight of daytime. Melatonin that doesn't shut off properly in the daytime is considered a cause of seasonal affective disorder syndrome ("winter depression" or SADS).

Dopamine: A mood-elevating chemical messenger produced in the brain and body; it is also important in sexual arousal, acts to prevent Parkinson's disease, and also functions as an inhibitory chemical messenger that participates in regulating milk secretion by the breast.

Down-regulation: A process in the brain and body in which the number (or function) of cell receptors are decreased. May occur as a natural process or due to medication effects. Example, in the second half of the menstrual cycle, progesterone down-regulates estradiol receptors.

Dyspareunia: medical term for vulvar and vaginal pain that occurs during penetration of the vagina, such as during sexual intercourse. A Vaginal dryness caused by loss of estradiol is a common cause that is treatable with topical estrogen tablets, rings and creams.

Endocrine Glands: Glands that manufacture and secrete hormones.

Endocrinologist: A medical specialist in diseases of the endocrine glands and their hormones; Endocrinology is the study and treatment of disorders of the glands and the hormones they secrete.

Endometrial Hyperplasia: Abnormal degree of thickening of the lining of the uterus, usually due to excess estrogen effect with insufficient progesterone or progestin effect. If left uncontrolled, over time the thickening of the lining can increase the risk of developing endometrial cancer.

Endometrial Lining: (also called Endometrium): the lining of the uterus. This tissue grows under the influence of estrogen (proliferative endometrium), and thickens under the influence of progesterone each month (secretory endometrium) in the menstrual cycle. When progesterone falls just before menses, or when you stop taking a progestin like Provera, Aygestin, Micronor, BCP, etc., it triggers a shedding of the secretory endometrium, which you experience as a menstrual bleeding.

Endometriosis: The presence of small islands (implants) of endometrium lying outside of the uterus, scattered about the abdomen and pelvic cavities and many times stuck on the outside of the intestine and bladder. Endometrium tissue is normally found only inside the uterus, and menstrual blood is released to the outside of the body via the vagina. When these implants bleed at the time of menses, they cause such severe pain because the blood is released into the abdomen and pelvis and acts as a significant irritant to other organs.

Enterohepatic Circulation: Blood flow from the gastrointestinal tract to the liver and that prolongs the action of compounds such as estrogen and other hormones by allowing them to "recirculate" rather than being excreted in the stool.

Endorphins (Also Enkephalins): natural pain-relieving and mood-elevating compounds (peptides) produced in the brain, spinal cord and body to produce a morphine-like analgesia.

Enzymes: Proteins produced by living cells that assist body functions by acting as catalysts in specific biochemical reactions. Enzyme catalysts are not themselves consumed in the reactions.

Epinephrine (Adrenaline): A chemical messenger made by the adrenal gland that prepares the body to handle emergencies called the "fight-or-flight" response. Epinephrine is also made in the laboratory to be used as a drug to treat severe allergic reactions, asthma, severe bleeding, and certain types of heart rhythm problems.

Equine Estrogens, Equilin: Estrogens derived from the pregnant mares' urine and used to make the animal-derived estrogen, Premarin®. These estrogens are chemically different from the ones made by the human ovary. They have some effects that are similar to human estrogens, and some effects that are quite different from human estrogens.

Essential Fatty Acids: Fatty acids necessary for cellular metabolism, which cannot be made by the body, but must be supplied in the diet. Good sources are fish oil, oils from nuts and seeds, and evening primrose oil.

Estrogen: The group of three sex hormones produced by the gonads (ovary in women, testes in men), and by the adrenal gland. In women, the higher amounts of these sex hormones are responsible for the female characteristics of breasts, feminine curves, menstruation, pregnancy.

    ❧ **Estrone (E1):** One of the human estrogens made by the ovary, adrenal gland and body fat before menopause. It is the one found in higher amounts after menopause because it is still made by body fat and to a lesser extent, the adrenal glands. Estrone serves as a "storage" form of estrogen for the ovary to make the more active estradiol before menopause. High estrone levels are more associated with breast and uterine cancers, a good reason to maintain a healthy percent body fat and weight.

    ❧ **Estradiol (E2, 17 beta estradiol):** The primary estrogen produced by the ovary before menopause. It is the biologically active estrogen at the estrogen receptors and the most potent of all the natural human estrogens. Estradiol is involved in over 400 functions in a woman's body, and is the form of estrogen that is lost at menopause when the ovary follicles are depleted.

    ❧ **Estriol (E3):** The weakest of the primary human estrogens, it is produced in large amounts during pregnancy. It is barely detectable in the nonpregnant female body, so women do not normally have estriol present to a measurable degree on a continuous basis and it has not been shown to have bone, heart or brain preserving effects.

> **Estradiol Valerate:** a more potent, synthetic estrogen, chemically different from the 17-beta estradiol produced by the ovary; used for menopausal hormone therapy in Europe for many years, but not used very often in the United States.

> **Ethinyl Estradiol:** a more potent synthetic estrogen used in birth control pills where the higher potency is needed (with the synthetic progestins) to adequately suppress the ovaries and provide reliable contraception. Not generally used in the United States for menopausal hormone therapy.

Fallopian Tubes: The tubes that carry the egg (ovum) from the ovary to the uterus. Fertilization of the egg occurs in the outer part of the fallopian tube.

Feedback: The process by which products made in a series of reactions provide messages back to the beginning of the process to control further reactions. Feedback may be electrical, chemical or mechanical, or thermal. Example of a thermal "feedback" is the thermostat that controls your furnace. Chemical feedback occurs with hormone levels reach a critical level and feed back to the brain that no more is needed for awhile.

Female Sex Hormones: The two sex hormones produced by the female ovary and placenta during pregnancy, estrogen (see above for types) and progesterone. Women's ovaries and adrenal glands also produce androgens, commonly referred to as "male" hormones, that are involved in many functions in a woman's body, including sexual desire and arousal.

Fertilization: The union of the female egg (ovum) with the male sperm (spermatozoa), which occurs in the fallopian tube.

Fetus: A developing human from the end of the eighth week of pregnancy until birth.

Fibrocystic: Development of dense, lumpy, ropy (fibrous) changes in tissue. About 60-70% of healthy women will have "fibrocystic" changes in their breasts, and this does not indicate a disease process. Similar changes may occur in muscle tissue in chronic pain syndromes.

Fibroids (Fibromas): Noncancerous growths of the uterus consisting of muscle and fibrous tissue. The medical term is leiomyoma, or sometimes just "myomas." The presence of fibroids tends to cause heavy, painful bleeding and cramps. At times they cause back pain, referred pain to the hip, or bladder pain and pressure with incontinence, depending on where the fibroids are found in the uterus.

Fibromyalgia: a syndrome of diffuse muscle pain and tender points, commonly triggered by imbalances of ovarian and thyroid hormones along with other causes.

First-pass Metabolism: Breakdown of chemicals, medications, hormones, etc. by the liver as a first-step after being absorbed into the bloodstream from the gastrointestinal tract. First-pass metabolism can eliminate as much as 70% or more of an oral dose of a medication or hormone. This step is omitted when medications and hormones are absorbed directly into the bloodstream from the skin (patch or cream) or muscle (injection).

Follicle Stimulating Hormone (FSH): A hormone secreted by the pituitary gland that reaches the ovaries via the blood circulation and stimulates the growth of ovarian follicles to form the egg that is released at ovulation. FSH above 10-15 when the brain senses a decline in ovarian hormones, and levels of FSH greater than 20 are defined as menopausal. FSH also functions in men to stimulate the sperm-producing cells in the testes; high FSH levels in men indicate low levels of testosterone, sometimes called "andropause."

Follicular (Phase): The first half of the ovarian hormone cycle leading up to the release of the egg at ovulation. Estrogen (estradiol) is the dominant hormone for this part of the cycle, and there is very little progesterone present.

Free Hormone: Hormone that is circulating in the bloodstream not connected to a carrier protein, and therefore "free" to be biologically active at cell receptor sites. See also "bound hormone."

Frigid (Sexual): A negative term applied to women who are considered by their partner to be sexually unresponsive and disinterested. Hormonal, medical, relationship, situational and lifestyle factors may cause loss of sexual desire and responsiveness, and all of these should be properly evaluated to determine the cause of sexual difficulties.

FSD: (Female Sexual Dysfunction): There are several different types and a variety of hormonal, medical, relationship, stress and other causes.

Galactorrhea: The presence of milk or milky fluid in the breasts when not breast-feeding. It is usually a symptom of elevated prolactin, which may be caused by some medications (such as antidepressants) or by benign hormone-producing tumors (adenomas) of the pituitary gland.

Gamma Aminobutyric Acid (GABA): an inhibitory neurotransmitter in the brain and nerves throughout the body; activation of this neurotransmitter produces a calming or anti-anxiety effect.

Gamma Linolenic Acid (GLA): An omega 6 essential fatty acid that is used to synthesize prostaglandins. It has an anti-inflammatory effect in the body. Good sources: breast milk, evening primrose oil, borage plant oil, and black currant seed oil.

Genistein: isoflavone compound (also called phytoestrogen) found in soy and other plants that has weak estrogen-like effects. In some concentrations it acts to block estrogen receptors, while in other concentrations it may stimulate the estrogen receptors in body tissues, including breast cancers.

Glands: Body organs or tissues, generally soft and fleshy in consistency, that manufacture and secrete or excrete hormones, chemicals that exert their effects on target organs elsewhere in the body.

Glucocorticoid (also called Corticosteroids): A group of hormones produced in the adrenal cortex that are primarily active in protecting against stress and in regulating protein and carbohydrate metabolism. These compounds (such as cortisone) tend to increase blood glucose, liver glycogen, and suppress the immune response and inflammatory response. Levels that are too high over time cause bone loss. See also Cushing's and Addison's disease.

Gynecology: Surgical specialty of medicine that provides surgical and medicinal treatments for problems related to women's reproductive organs.

Half-life: A measurement of how long it takes for half of a substance to be lost or removed; for example, drug half-life refers to how long it takes for the concentration of a drug or hormone to be decreased by one-half due to metabolic break-down or excretion. It is usually estimated that it takes five half-lives for a drug or other substance to be completely gone from the body.

HDL: see cholesterol

Hirsutism: A condition of excessive facial and body hair (excluding hair on the scalp) and often in women is due to excess of androgens.

Hormones: Chemicals produced by various glands that are then transported around the body to exert their multiple metabolic effects.

Hormone Receptor Site: A "binding" or "docking" site in or on cells for hormones to connect in order to exert their actions. The hormone and its receptor create what is called a "receptor complex" that sends signals to the cell to carry out various functions.

Hormone Replacement Therapy (HRT): Technically, the administration of any hormonal preparations (natural or synthetic) to replace the loss of natural hormones produced by various glands (thyroid, ovary, testes, pancreas, adrenal, pituitary, etc.). HRT in common usage now refers to administration of female hormones (estrogen and progestin) after menopause.

Hot Flash (Flush): Episode of vasodilation in skin of head, neck, and chest, accompanied by sensation of suffocation, sweating, feeling suddenly hot or cold. Occurs commonly during menopause due to falling hormone levels that trigger changes in the brain heat regulatory center.

HSD (Hypoactive Sexual Desire): diminished or absent interest in sexual activities, thoughts and fantasies. If it is accompanied by personal distress about this loss, it is considered a disorder (HSDD).

Hyperthyroidism: A condition caused by excessive hormone secretion of the thyroid glands that will increase the basal metabolic rate, increase heart rate and blood pressure, disrupt sleep, and may cause marked weight loss.

Hypoestrogenic: The condition of having less than optimal levels of estradiol from any cause. Estradiol decline leads to classic symptoms affecting many different body systems, such as hot flashes, insomnia, memory loss, headaches, palpitations, fatigue, thinning hair, dry skin/eyes, bone loss, rise in cholesterol and blood pressure, urinary leakage, loss of libido, vaginal dryness, muscle aches, crawly skin, etc.

Hypothalamus: The "master conductor" or "control center" situated at the base of the brain regulates body temperature, thirst, appetite, sex drive, and all other hormonal glands. It releases hormones that travel directly to the pituitary gland and stimulate the release of pituitary hormones, which govern the other endocrine glands.

Hypothyroidism: A slowing of overall body metabolism due to deficiency of the thyroid hormone production or function. There are many diverse symptoms, but common ones include obesity, dry skin and hair, low blood pressure, slow pulse, sluggishness of all functions, constipation, depressed mood, muscle aches/weakness, hair loss, low energy, goiter.

Hysterectomy: Surgical removal (abdominal or vaginal) of the uterus only. In common usage, women may say "hysterectomy" when both the uterus and ovaries have been removed or when just the uterus has been removed. The medical term for removal of the uterus and ovaries together is "hysterectomy with bilateral salpingo-oophorectomy (BSO)".

Immune System: The defense and surveillance system of the body that protects against infection by micro-organisms and invasion by foreign tissues and substances. The immune system is made up of specialized blood cells (lymphocytes, B-cells, T-cells, etc.), blood proteins (antibodies), the spleen, thymus gland, lymph nodes, bone marrow. Immune function is impaired with a variety of endocrine imbalances, such as decline in ovarian hormones, thyroid and adrenal disorders.

Implant: A device that is surgically implanted into a part of the body for cosmetic or therapeutic purposes. Hormone-containing implants are sometimes used for contraception or for menopausal hormone replacement therapy.

Inflammation: A condition characterized by swelling, redness, heat, and pain in any tissue as a result of trauma, irritation, infection, or imbalances in immune function. A high level of C-reactive protein (CRP-hs) is a general marker in the bloodstream indicating the presence of inflammation of any kind.

Insulin: A hormone secreted by beta cells of the pancreas that is essential for the proper metabolism of blood sugar (glucose), for maintenance of proper blood sugar level, and for promoting storage of fat. Insulin medication is used to control high blood sugar in diabetes.

Isoflavone: Chemical compounds found in a variety of plants (soy, red clover, etc.) that are weakly estrogenic in their effects and are often called phytoestrogens (phyto meaning derived from plants). Common isoflavones that are being studied for their health effects are genistein, daidzein, biochanin, and formononetin. Many of these compounds can inhibit the effects of the body's natural ovarian hormones and should be used cautiously in pre-menopausal women, especially if trying to become pregnant.

IUD: Intrauterine device, an object inserted into the uterus, typically used for contraception, but may also be a means of delivering hormones (example: Mirena progestin delivery system).

Kegel Exercises: isolation and repeated intentional contraction and relaxation of the muscles that control urinary flow to strengthen the muscles and help prevent urinary leakage and enhance pleasure during sexual activity.

Laparoscope: A long thin telescopic instrument utilizing a fiberoptic lighting system, which is inserted through a small incision in the abdominal wall. It functions like a hollow flashlight enabling the surgeon to view internal organs and insert operating instruments through its hollow tube.

LDL: see cholesterol.

Libido: Level of sexual desire or sex drive, sexual energy, or motivation and interest in sexual activity.

Lichen Sclerosus: thinning or atrophy of vulvar tissues that can cause persistent itching and dryness, as well as pain during sexual activity. Cream forms of estradiol and testosterone are often used to treat this condition.

Lipoproteins: carrier proteins in the bloodstream that transport fats (cholesterol and triglycerides) in the blood.

Luteal (Phase): The progesterone-dominant second half of the menstrual cycle, from ovulation until menses begin. The primary hormone of this phase is progesterone that is the primary hormone trigger for "PMS."

Luteinizing Hormone (LH): A hormone produced by the pituitary gland that triggers ovulation and the egg release to become the corpus luteum. In men, LH stimulates production of testosterone by the testes and LH levels will rise in men with low testosterone.

Male Hormone: A hormone in the androgen group that promotes masculine characteristics in the body such as facial and body hair pattern, acne, deepening of the voice, increased muscle mass, and increased libido. At lower levels, these hormones play important roles in healthy function of many systems for women. See androgen.

Malignant: cancer, cancerous.

Manic Depression (Bipolar Disorder): A biological disorder of brain function that produces episodes of euphoria, delusions, and abnormally increased energy, alternating at variable intervals with severe depressions.

Melatonin: A hormone produced by the pineal gland in the brain and is involved in regulating the sleep-wake cycle; levels rise during darkness and fall at daylight. Excess melatonin levels that fail to shut off during the day have been thought to cause seasonal affective disorder (SADS).

Menopause: The cessation of menstruation. The last period. May be natural (due to depletion of the ovarian follicles) or surgical removal of the uterus (without or with removal of ovaries). Premature menopause can also be caused by illnesses, medications and toxins that damage the ovaries. When the ovaries are gone or have lost their follicles, the body loses the hormones estradiol, progesterone, testosterone and much of the DHEA. The period of time leading up the menopause, when hormone production by the ovaries is decreasing, is called the climacteric.

Menstrual Clock: A specialized part of the hypothalamus regulating the cyclical timing of the phases of the menstrual cycle.

Menstruation: Monthly bleeding from the vagina in women from puberty until menopause, caused by shedding of the lining of the womb (uterus) if there is no fertilization of an egg.

Metabolic Hormones: Hormones that are involved in regulating cellular energy processes, synthesis of body proteins, and other functions involved in tissue growth and repair.

Metabolic Rate: The rate at which the body converts chemical energy in foods into heat (thermal) and movement (kinetic) energy. Metabolic rate is governed by hormones from the thyroid, ovary, testes, adrenal, and pancreas.

Metabolism: Chemical processes, regulated by hormones, utilizing the raw materials of food nutrients, oxygen, minerals, vitamins along with enzymes to produce energy for body functions such as growth, repair, healing. See also anabolic, catabolic metabolism

Metabolite: Any product of metabolism. Some metabolites are active and needed for other functions, and some metabolites may be toxic and need to be excreted. An example of a toxic metabolite is ammonia from the breakdown of protein; an active metabolite of progesterone has anxiety-relieving properties when it binds to the brain's GABA receptor.

Microgram: One-millionth part of a gram. One thousandth of a milligram. The abbreviation on prescriptions is mcg.

Micronized: to make into small particles in the micron size range.

Milligram: One-thousandth of a gram. The abbreviation on prescriptions is mg. See also picogram, nanogram

Milliliter: One-thousandth of a liter, or about 1 cc. The abbreviation on prescriptions is ml.

Mineralocorticoid: Hormones, such as aldosterone, that is produced by the adrenal gland and functions to regulate electrolytes (sodium, potassium, chloride) and water balance in the body.

Molecule: A chemical compound made up of different arrangements and types of atoms; a molecule is the smallest unit into which a substance may be divided without loss of its unique characteristics.

Myomectomy: surgical removal of fibroids (myomas) but leaving the uterus and cervix intact. This procedure preserves fertility, but frequently may become a more complicated surgery with greater blood loss than hysterectomy. Complications and risk of damage may be similar to hysterectomy. Careful evaluation by an experienced surgeon is important to determine whether is woman is a good candidate for myomectomy.

Nanogram: One billionth of a gram, abbreviated as ng.

"Natural" Hormone: Bioidentical hormones are often called "natural" hormones, but "natural" may also refer to a biological source (such as the horse) that produces molecules different from those made by the human body. Bioidentical is a more correct term than "natural" when referring to the types made by the human body and pharmaceuticals that are designed to duplicate ones made by the body. Hormones that are "bio-identical" may be made in the laboratory from building blocks found in plants, but end up with the same chemical structure as the hormones made by body organs such as the thyroid and ovary.

Neuron: A nerve cell, the structure and functional unit of the nervous system. Neurons function in initiation and conduction of electrical and chemical "nerve" impulses.

Neurotransmitters: Chemicals that transmit messages from nerve cell to nerve cell in the brain, and between the brain and the tissues and organs of the body. Common ones referred to throughout this book are serotonin, dopamine, acetylcholine, GABA, norepinephrine.

Non-androgenic: Not causing masculine hormone effects in the body.

Norepinephrine (Noradrenaline): A hormone produced by the adrenal gland, and certain areas of the brain that helps the body prepare for and cope with stress. It also has a mood-elevating effect, but levels that are too high may cause feelings of anxiety, raise blood pressure and cause insomnia. Epinephrine (Adrenaline) is another "stress-hormone" produced by the adrenal gland with similar effects in some tissues and opposite effects in yet others.

Nucleus: The vital body inside cells that contains the genetic material (DNA) and is responsible for regulation of essential functions for cell growth, protein synthesis, metabolism, reproduction, and transmission of characteristics of a cell.

Oophorectomy (Ovariectomy): Surgical removal of the ovaries.

Oral: Indicating something is to be taken by mouth.

Orgasm: The physical and emotional release of tension following sexual arousal; also called climax.

Osteoblast: Cells that function to build new bone. These cells are stimulated by estradiol, testosterone and to a lesser extent, progesterone.

Osteoclast: Cells that are responsible for resorption (breaking down) old brittle bone. Their action is regulated primarily by estradiol and testosterone to a lesser extent.

Osteopenia: Loss of bone density that is not yet severe enough to be considered osteoporosis. Osteopenia will progress to osteoporosis if active measures are not taken to maintain bone (such as calcium, magnesium, exercise, and hormone therapy).

Osteoporosis: Loss of bone density (mass) due to loss of bone minerals and reduction of the normal bony architecture that provides strength to the skeleton. Causes bones to become porous, brittle and more easily broken.

Ova (Ovum): An ovarian follicle that has released to become the egg (ova) at ovulation. A ova that is fertilized with sperm becomes an embryo that develops into a fetus.

Ovaries: The female sex glands (gonads) located on each side of the uterus, which produce eggs and the female sex hormones (estrogen and progesterone), along with testosterone and DHEA.

Ovulation: The release of the egg from the ovary occurring around mid-cycle.

Ovulation Pain: "Mittelschmerz" pain occurring at ovulation, which may be sharp and severe and last from a few minutes up to twelve hours.

Pancreas: A gland situated behind the stomach that produces pancreatic juice (contains digestive enzymes such as lipase and amylase) and also the hormones insulin and glucagon that function to regulate blood sugar and carbohydrate metabolism.

Parasympathetic Nervous System: The part of the autonomic nervous system that regulates body relaxation and functions of growth and repair such as digestion. Its primary chemical messenger or neurotransmitter is acetylcholine.

Parenteral: A method of delivering substances (such as medications) directly to the bloodstream bypassing the digestive system and liver metabolism. Parenteral routes include: vaginal and rectal suppositories/tablets, sublingual tablets/capsules, transdermal (skin patch), subcutaneous (implant), intramuscular (IM) and intravenous (IV) injections. All of these avoid the "first-pass" hepatic (liver) metabolism.

Peak Level: The highest level of a hormone or medication that is reached after taking a dose or being produced by the body. ("Trough" level is the lowest point reached after a medication or hormone is taken or produced by the body).

Pelvic Inflammatory Disease (PID): Inflammation of the pelvic organs, particularly the uterus and fallopian tubes, caused by infectious micro-organisms, typically occurring from sexually-transmitted bacteria, fungi, and viruses. PID typically causes pain, and can also cause damage to the ovaries, resulting in decreased hormone production

Perimenopausal: Time frame of several years prior to menopause when menstrual periods start to be skipped and continuing through menopause to the first few years just after periods stop. It has a variable age of onset and symptoms commonly include insomnia, mood changes, bone loss, cholesterol changes, disrupted sleep, hot flashes, and other phenomena. (See also premenopausal)

Pharmacokinetics/Dynamics: Study of drug absorption, delivery to tissues of the body, metabolism and excretion.

Physiological: Normal body processes and functions.

Phytoestrogens: Plant(phyto) derived chemical molecules that may attach to the body's estrogen receptors and trigger certain estrogen-like actions; some of these compounds have estrogen-blocking actions (antagonists) that may cause decreased production of the body's own ovarian hormones in premenopausal women. Occur naturally in several hundred different types of plants, including soy, clover and a variety of grains.

Picogram: One trillionth of a gram, abbreviated pg.

Pituitary Gland: A mushroom-shaped gland connected by a vascular stalk to the base of the brain. The pituitary gland manufactures hormones (FSH, LH, TSH, ACTH, and others) that in turn control other hormonal glands, such as the thyroid, adrenals, ovaries, and breasts.

Placenta: The hormonal organ designed to provide for the nourishment of the fetus and the elimination of its waste products. It produces a number of hormones, such as progesterone, estriol and others that have roles in sustaining pregnancy and adapting the mother's body to adjust to the increased physiological demands of pregnancy. It is formed in the uterus by the union of uterine mucous membrane with membranes of the fetus

Plaque: A deposit of platelets, fibrin, calcium, cholesterol and other fatty substances that build up in arteries and cause clogging that leads to reduced blood flow and may cause angina, heart attacks, or strokes. The whole process of plaque build-up and artery damage is referred to as atherosclerosis.

Plasma: The liquid part of blood and the lymph (minus the red and white blood cells) that contains proteins, clotting factors, and other chemicals such as glucose, hormones, etc.

PMS: see Premenstrual Syndrome.

Polycystic Ovary Syndrome (PCO): A hereditary disorder of the ovaries in which the usual female hormonal balance is altered, and there are excessive levels of insulin and male hormones accompanied by changes in body shape, irregular menstruation and infertility. It may also be triggered by exposure to environmental endocrine disrupter chemicals, severe stress, marked weight gain, or chronic use of herbs that interfere with ovarian function. In PCO syndrome, the ovaries have multiple small follicles or "cysts," which can be sometimes, but not always, be seen on an ultrasound scan of the pelvis. Other common features: truncal obesity, acne, thinning of scalp hair, excess body hair, mood swings, glucose intolerance and insulin resistance, hypertension, and increased risk of diabetes and early-onset heart disease.

Post-menopause: The years following the end of menstruation and decline in production of ovarian female hormones (menopause).

Postnatal, Post-partum: The time period after childbirth.

Precursor: A substance ("building block") that is used to make another compound, hormone or medication. For example, cholesterol molecules are used as the precursor building blocks for the body to make other steroid hormones, such as progesterone, estradiol and testosterone.

Premature Menopause: Cessation of menses and decline of ovarian hormone production occurring before the age of forty-two.

Pre-menopausal: The time leading up to menopause characterized by hormonal changes and irregular menstrual flow. It may begin as much as ten years before actual menopause, but more commonly occurs about four to five years before menopause (see also perimenopause).

PreMenstrual Syndrome (PMS): A collection of variable symptoms such as mood disturbance, headaches, abdominal bloating, etc. recurring on a cyclical basis in the week or two before menstrual bleeding (see also perimenopause).

Progesterone: A steroid hormone produced by the corpus luteum (formed from the egg released at ovulation in the ovary) or placenta during pregnancy. Small amounts are also made by the adrenal glands. Responsible for secretory changes in uterine endometrium in second half of menstrual cycle to prepare the uterus to receive and nourish a fertilized egg. Progesterone also has many metabolic functions designed help a mother's body change in ways that will support a pregnancy (pro-gestation hormone = progesterone).

Progestin: A group of hormones that have progesterone-like effects on the uterus and body; progesterone is correctly included in this larger class of hormones, but common usage usually means that "progestin" refers to synthetic compounds that are made in the laboratory and chemically different from the natural ovary hormone progesterone.

Progestin-only Pill ("mini-pill"): A contraceptive pill containing only a progestin such as norethindrone (Brands: Micronor, Nor QD, and others). Unless it is given with estrogen to balance the unwanted side effects, the progestin-only pills are not recommended for midlife women due to the potential for adverse effects on cholesterol, glucose control and body weight. Progestin-only pills, implants or injections are not recommended for women with a history of depression, diabetes, headaches, hypertension or weight gain as progestins aggravate all of these problems unless estrogen is also given.

Progestogens: Natural or synthetic substances that have effects similar to the natural female hormone progesterone. Synthetic progestogens (called progestins) are commonly used in birth control pills and HRT to regulate menstrual bleeding. Examples are medroxyprogesterone acetate (Provera, Cycrin), norethindrone (Aygestin, Micronor), norethisterone, norgestrel, levonorgestrel (in Mirena and many birth control pills), drospirenone (in Yasmin), etonongestrel (in Nuvaring), and others.

Prolactin: A hormone secreted by the pituitary gland that stimulates milk production in the breasts. At times other than nursing, high levels of prolactin may cause headaches, weight gain, depression and breast discharge (galactorrhea).

Prostaglandins: Chemicals manufactured throughout the body that exert a hormone-like effect and influence muscular (including the uterus) contraction, circulation, and inflammation. Release of prostaglandins in the uterus when progesterone falls at the time of menstruation is a cause of menstrual cramps.

Psychosis: A severe biochemical disorder of brain function characterized by delusions, hallucinations, and abnormalities in thinking and reasoning. It may be due to many causes: schizophrenia, major depression, manic-depressive disorder, alcohol intoxication, severe endocrine illness (example: hyper and hypothyroidism), drug abuse (cocaine), and medication toxicity (such as atropine, digitalis, lidocaine, stimulants and many others).

Psychosomatic: Physical symptoms that are triggered by psychological and emotional causes and not due primarily to physical disease. This term is often misused when applied to women, as in "the cause isn't known so it must be psychosomatic, or stress-related."

Psychotherapy: The process of using systematic "talking" approaches to treat stress-related problems, emotional issues, and disturbances in self-image. Many different methods may be used, depending upon the training of the therapist.

Psychotropic Drugs: Drugs that act primarily on the brain to produce effects on mood, thinking, sleep, and other functions. Examples are sedatives, tranquilizers (anti-anxiety agents), anti-depressants, anti-psychotics, analgesic and anesthetic agents.

Puerperium: The period of time after childbirth required to return the reproductive organs to their prepregnant size and condition. This takes six to eight weeks.

Receptor: see hormone receptor.

Receptor Antagonist (Blocker): A compound, hormone or medication that binds at a cell's receptor site but blocks the normal action of that receptor system. Examples are "beta-blockers" that block the normal action of the beta adrenergic receptors; tamoxifen that blocks the estrogen receptor of the breast and brain even though it will activate the estrogen receptors in the uterine lining (endometrium).

Rectal: Pertaining to the rectum.

Sebaceous Glands: The tiny oil-producing glands in the skin. If they overproduce oil and/or become obstructed, pimples or acne will result.

Sensate Focus: a series of intimate exercises to enhance sexual pleasuring. See discussion in text for stages of Sensate Focus exercises.

SERMS: An abbreviation for a class of medications called Selective Estrogen Receptor Modulators. These drugs have both agonist (activating) and antagonist (blocking) actions at the body's estrogen receptors, depending on the particular organ. Examples are tamoxifen and raloxifen; both drugs block breast estrogen receptors, and stimulate estrogen receptors elsewhere (such as bone). Because they block important actions of estrogen, they are not a pure replacement for all of estrogen's actions in the body. Side effects of both medicines include hot flashes, formation of blood clots, pulmonary emboli, cataracts, and increased risk of uterine cancer (tamoxifen).

Serotonin (5-HT): A potent brain chemical that regulates sleep, mood, libido, appetite, pain, and repetitive thoughts and actions. Serotonin's chemical name is 5-hydroxytryptophan and it is made by the brain and body from dietary sources of the amino acid tryptophan (milk, turkey, whole grains, etc.).

Serum: The fluid portion of the blood after coagulation has removed the cells, fibrin and fibrinogen.

Sex Hormones: The male and female hormones produced from cholesterol by the testicles, ovaries, adrenal glands, and body fat: testosterone, estrogens, progesterone, androgens.

Sex Hormone Binding Globulin: A carrier protein in the bloodstream (made in the liver) that binds or carries estrogen, testosterone, progesterone to provide a reservoir of hormones ready for release into the free fraction to become the active form.

Sex therapy: a form of non-hormonal, non-medical talk therapy (psychotherapy) used by qualified practitioners to treat a variety of sexual problems and relationship issues affecting sexual activity.

Steroid Drugs and Hormones: The group of chemical substances that has a chemical structure consisting of multiple rings of carbon atoms. Examples include estrogen, progesterone, and testosterone (sex hormones), cortisol (hormone), Cortisone (the drug).

Stress (Urinary) Incontinence: Loss of urine due to pressure on weakened bladder structures and supporting ligaments; this weakness occurs as a result of estrogen loss and damage during childbirth. Increased pressure on the bladder may come from coughing, sneezing, laughing, straining to lift objects, or prolonged standing.

Stroke: Brain damage resulting from diminished blood supply and oxygen (ischemia) to the brain; usually occurs as a result of a clot blocking the arteries.

Sublingual: Something (medication, hormones, allergy drops, etc.) given underneath the tongue to be absorbed into the blood stream.

Sustained (Timed) Release: A process in which a medication is prepared or formulated in such a way as to deliver small amounts over a longer period of time.

Sympathetic Nervous System: The part of the autonomic nervous system that prepares the body for stress through effects of the stress hormones it releases (examples: by increasing oxygen to the tissues, increasing heart rate, blood pressure and glucose release, etc.). Its primary chemical messengers (neurotransmitters) are norepinephrine and epinephrine.

Symptoms: Any physical or emotional change in the body that is perceived as distressing or painful. "Symptom" usually means a change that makes a person feel unwell. "Phenomena" is a word used to describe changes that don't necessarily cause distress.

Syndrome: A group of symptoms and objective signs that typically occur together and serve to characterize a disease or disorder.

Synergistic: Substances interacting in ways that produce an effect greater than just adding the effects of the combined substances.

Synthetic: Made by synthesis; can be identical to a natural compound found in the body, or may be synthesized to be chemically different and have different properties. Synthetic simply means "made by synthesis", it does not mean "artificial" (although common usage often implies "artificial" when the term synthetic is used to apply to a hormone).

Testes: The male gonads; two reproductive glands located in the scrotum that produce the male reproductive cells or spermatozoa and the male hormone, testosterone.

Testosterone: The major male sex hormone produced in the testes and also produced by the female ovary; plays major role in men and women for sexual desire and arousal, maintaining bone and muscle mass, cognitive function, and psychological well-being.

Thyroid Gland: The endocrine gland situated in front of the larynx that produces the major hormones of metabolism; thyroxine (T4) and tri-iodothyronine (T3); also produces calcitonin that regulates calcium balance.

Thyroid Stimulating Hormone (TSH): The hormone produced by the brain that regulates the production and release of thyroid hormones from the thyroid gland. TSH levels are low in hyperthyroidism, and high in hypothyroidism.

Trandermal: absorbed through the skin into the bloodstream from a cream or patch or injection; this form of delivery bypasses the liver's "first-pass" metabolism.

Triglycerides (TG): One of the blood fats that the body can use to make cholesterol; elevated TG (from diet, alcohol intake, lack of exercise, and some drugs) are a significant and independent risk factor for heart disease in women and also increase the risk of diabetes. Consists of one glycerol and three fatty acids.

Tryptophan: An amino acid found in foods that is the major precursor ("building block") for the body and brain to make serotonin (5-hydroxytryptophan, 5-HT).

Tubal Ligation (BTL): The surgical procedure to cut or tie the fallopian tubes and prevent "eggs" released from the ovary from reaching the uterus. BTL is used as a method of contraception, considered permanent because it is difficult and expensive to reverse, with low probability of success. Some women notice "worsening PMS" and other symptoms of imbalance or decrease in ovarian hormones after tubal ligation, and this is likely due to diminished blood flow to the ovaries from the procedure.

Tumor: An abnormal growth; may be cancerous or benign. An example is a uterine fibroid, a benign abnormal growth in the uterus (see Fibroid).

Up-regulation: the process of increasing the number or function of cellular receptors.

Urethra: A muscular tube that carries urine from the bladder to the outside of the body. Inflammation of this tube is called urethritis, and causes painful, burning sensations on urination.

Uterus: The womb or female reproductive organ that carries and nourishes a growing fetus; made up of an inner layer (see endometrium above), and a thick muscular layer that undergoes rhythmic contractions during labor and delivery, during menstruation, and during orgasm (although not all women feel this).

Urologist: A surgeon who specializes in diseases of the kidneys, urinary tract and bladder.

Ultrasound Scan: A method of using very high frequency sound waves to visualize internal organs, blood vessels, and the fetus in pregnancy. The sound waves used are more than 20,000 hertz, and above the level that humans can hear. Ultrasound images do not involve using radiation sources, so there is no exposure to radiation during the procedure.

Vagina: The "birth canal" or genital passage leading from the uterus to the outside of the body at the vulva; it is muscular and elastic, expanding to accommodate the penis during intercourse, or to accommodate a baby during delivery.

Vaginal Ring: a small, soft plastic or silastic device containing hormones or other medication for direct topical delivery to the vagina and urinary system. An example is Estring, containing 17-beta estradiol, used to treat vaginal dryness.

Vaginismus: involuntary, painful spasms of the muscles around the entry of the vagina causing pain with attempted penetration during sexual activity.

Vasoactive Hormone or Drugs: Drugs or substances acting on the blood vessels to cause either dilation (example: estradiol, nitroglycerine) or constriction (example: nicotine) of the arteries.

Vasomotor: A term that refers to the way that nerve cells connect at the smooth muscle wall of arteries and govern the opening (vasodilation) and closing (vasoconstriction) of blood vessels to control blood flow.

Virilization: The development of masculine physical characteristics due to presence of male hormones. Virilization may occur in women if the androgen hormones are too high.

Vulva: Female external genitalia. Also known as the lips of the vaginal opening.

Vulvar Vestibulitis: inflammation and burning pain around the opening to the vagina, often causing pain with daily activities as well as during sex.

Vulvodynia: burning pain, with or without itching, affecting the external genital tissue called the vulva. May have many causes, in particular, the loss of estradiol as women approach menopause.

Wild (Mexican) Yam: A root vegetable that grows in many areas and contains precursor compounds that can be extracted and used in the laboratory as building blocks to make the hormones estradiol, testosterone and progesterone. Extracts of wild yam cannot be converted by the human body to the human forms of active hormones, since we do not have the enzymes to carry out these chemical reactions.

Appendix II
Bibliography and Resources

It is not possible to list the hundreds of medical and scientific peer-reviewed articles from reputable medical journals that I have read and studied for my clinical work and this book. This is a list of selected *historical* and *current* articles that may be of interest for those of you who want a reference for your physician, or for your own reading of the medical literature. I have included older articles to illustrate how long this information has been available and how our current understandings have evolved from this historical foundation. Many of the concepts I described in this book have been described in the medical literature, but ignored, for decades. The current research articles help you see the depth and breadth of our existing science explaining these important hormone connections to the healthy function of our entire body. Each article provides additional references if you wish to pursue a topic in more depth.

For this book, I have focused on medical research articles published in the major, peer-reviewed national and international medical journals. I have also included a list of several national organizations that can be helpful resources for further information.

For additional information about important hormone connections in women's health, and more resources, you may find it helpful to read my other three books: *It's My Ovaries, Stupid!*, Scribner, New York, 2003; *Women, Weight and Hormones*, M. Evans, New York, 2001, and *Screaming to Be Heard: Hormone Connections Women Suspect and Doctors Still Ignore*, Revised Edition, M. Evans, New York, 2001.

I. Medical Bibliography

Abraham GE. Ovarian and adrenal contributions to peripheral androgens during the menstrual cycle. J Clin Endocrinol Metab 1974;39:340-6

Allolio B, Arlt W. DHEA treatment: myth or reality? Trends Endocrinol Metab. 2002 7:288-94.

Alder EM, Cook A, Davidson D, et al. Hormones, mood and sexuality in lactating women. Br J Psychiatry 1986;148:74-9

Aloia, J.F., McGowan, D.M., Vaswani, A.N., Ross, P. and Cohn, S.H. Relationship of menopause to skeletal and muscle mass. *Am. J. Clin. Nutr.*, (1991) 53, 1378-83

Anderson KE, Sellers TA, Chen PL, et al. Association of Stein-Leventhal syndrome with the incidence of postmenopausal breast carcinoma in a large prospective study of women in Iowa. Cancer 1997;79:494-99

Appelt H, Appelt SB. The psychoendocrinology of female sexuality. German J. Psychology 1986;10:143-56

Arlt W, Callies F, et. Al. Dehydroepiandrosterone replacement in women with adrenal insufficiency. New Engl J Med 2002; 341;1013-1020

Avis NE, Stellato R, Crawford S, Johannes C, Longcope C. Is there an association between menopause status and sexual functioning? *Menopause* 2000;7:297-309.

Bachman G, Bancroft J, Braunstein G, Burger H, Davis S, Dennerstein L, Goldstein I, Guay A, Leiblum S, Lobo R, Notelovitz M, Rosen R, Sarrel P, Sherwin B, Simon J, Simpson E, Shifren J, Spark R, Traish A. Female androgen insufficiency: the Princeton consensus statement on definition, classification, and assessment. Fertility and Sterility 2002; 77: 660-665.

Bachmann GA,Leiblum SR.The impact of hormones on menopausal sexuality: a literature review. *Menopause* 2004;11:120-130.

Backstrom CT, Boyle H, Baird DT. Persistence of symptoms of premenstrual tension in hysterectomized women. *Br J Obstet Gynaecol* 1981; 88:530-536.

Bale P, Doust J, Dawson D. Gymnasts, distance runners, anorexics body composition and menstrual status. *J Sports Med Phys Fitness.* 36(1):49-53, 1996.

Bancroft J, Cawood EHH. Androgens and the menopause: a study of 40-60 year-old women. Clin Endocrinol 1996;45:577-87

Bancroft J, Sanders D, Davidson D, Warner P. Mood, sexuality, hormones and the menstrual cycle III: Sexuality and the role of androgens. Psychosom Med 45; 509, 1983

Bancroft J, Sherwin B, Alexander GM, et al. Oral contraceptives, androgens, and the sexuality of young women, II: The role of androgens. Arch Sex Behav 1991;20:121-35

Bancroft, J., Sanders, D., Warner, P. and Loudon, N. The effects of oral contraceptives on mood and sexuality: comparison of triphasic and combined preparations. *J. Psychosom. Obstet. Gynaecol.*, 7, 1-8 1987

Barnhart KT, Freeman E, Grisso JA, et al. The effect of dehydroepiandrosterone supplementation to symptomatic perimenopausal women on serum endocrine profiles, lipid parameters, and health related quality of life. J Clin Endocrinol Metab 1999;84:3896-902

Barrett-Connor E, Young R, Notelovitz M, et al. A two-year, double-blind comparison of estrogen-androgen and conjugated estrogens in surgically menopausal women. J Reprod Med 1999;44:1012-20

Basson R. Female sexual response: the role of drugs in the management of sexual dysfunction.*Obstet Gynecol* .2001;98:350-353.

Basson R. Sexuality and sexual disorders.*Clinical Updates in Women 's Health Care* .2003;11:1-94.

Basson R, Berman J, Burnett A, et al. Report of the international consensus development conference on female sexual dysfunction:definitions and classifications.*J Urol* .2000;163:888-893.

Basson R,Leiblum S,Brotto L,et al. Definitions of women 's sexual dysfunction reconsidered: advocating expansion and revision. *J Psychosom Obstet Gynaecol* .2003;24:221-229.

Becker U, Tonnesen H, et al. Menstrual disturbances and fertility in chronic alcoholic women. IN: Drug and Alcohol Dependence, 24 (1989) 75-82, Elsevier Scientific Publishers Ireland

Berga SL. Stress and ovarian function. *Am J Sports Med.* 24(6 Suppl):S36-7, 1996.

Bhatia SK, Moore D, and Kalkhoff RK. Progesterone suppression of the plasma growth hormone Response. *J. Clin Endocrinol Metab* 35: 364-369; 1972.

Bloch M, Schmidt PJ, Danaceau M et al. Effects of gonadal steroids in women with a history of postpartum depression. *Am J Psychiatry* 157(6): 924-930, 2000.

Braunstein GD. Androgen insufficiency in women: summary of critical issues. Fertil Steril 2002;77:S94-S9

Brincat M, Studd JWW, O'Dowd T, et al. Subcutaneous hormone implants for the control of climacteric symptoms. *The Lancet* 1984;1:16-18

Brinton, RD and Nilsen J. Impact of progestins on estrogen-induced neuroprotection: synergy by progesterone and 19-norprogesterone and antagonism by medroxyprogesterone acetate. *Endocrinology* 143:2050212, 2002.

Bullen B, Skrinar G, Beitins I, et al. Endurance training effects on plasma hormonal responsiveness and sex hormone excretion. *J. Appl Phys: Respirat. Environ.Exercise Physiol* 1984; 56-6: l453-1463

Burger HG, Dudley EC, Cui J, et al. A prospective longitudinal study of serum testosterone, dehydroepiandrosterone sulfate, and sex hormone-binding globulin levels through the menopause transition. *J Clin Endodrinal Metab* 2000; 85:2832-8

Burger HG, Hailes J, Nelson J. Effect of combined implants of oestradiol and testosterone on libido in post-menopausal women. *Br Med J* 1987;294:936-7

Burger HG, Hailes J, Menelaus M, et al. The management of persistent menopausal symptoms with oestradiol testosterone implants: clinical, lipid and hormonal results. *Maturitas* 1984;6:351-8

Buster JE,Casson PR.Where androgens come from, what controls them, and whether to replace them. In: Lobo RA (Ed). *Treatment of the Postmenopausal-Woman*, Lippincott-Raven,1999, Philadelphia,PA

Buster JE, Casson PR, Straughn AB, et al. Postmenopausal steroid replacement with micronized dehydroepiandrosterone: preliminary oral bioavailability and dose proportionality studies. *Am J Obstet Gynecol* 1992;166:1163–1170.

Buvat J. Androgen therapy with dehydroepiandrosterone. *World J Urol.* 2003 5;346-55.

Cameron DR, Braunstein GD. Androgen replacement therapy in women. *Fertil Steril* 2004; 82: 273-289.

Casson PR, Carson SA, Buster JE, et al. Replacement dehydroepiandrosterone in elderly: rationale and prospects for the future. *Endocrinologist* 1998; 8:187–194.

Casson PR, Santoro NF, Elkind-Hirsch K, et al, Postmenopausal dehydroepiandrosterone (DHEA) administration increases free insulin-like growth factor-I (IGF-I) and decreases high density lipoprotein (HDL): a six month trial. *Fertil Steril* 1998;70:107–110.

Castracane, V.D., Stewart, D.R., Gimpel, T. *et al.* (1998) Maternal serum androgens in human pregnancy: early increases within the cycles of conception. *Hum. Reprod.*, **13**, 460–464.

Cawood EHH, Bancroft J. Steroid hormones, the menopause, sexuality and well-being of women. *Psycholog Med* 1996;26:925-36

Chang RJ, et al. Diagnosis of polycystic ovary syndrome. *Endocrinol Metab Clin North Am.* 28(2):397-408, vii.1999.

Chen EC, Brzyski RG. Exercise and reproductive dysfunction. *Fertil Steril.* 71(1):1-6, 1999.

Chlebowski RT, Hendrix SL, Langer RD, et al. Influence of estrogen plus progestin on breast cancer and mammography in healthy postmenopausal women: the Women's Health Initiative randomize3d trial. *JAMA* 2003;289:3243-3253

Cooper GS, Baird DD, Hulka BS, et al. Follicle-stimulating hormone concentrations in relation to active and passive smoking. *Obstet Gynecol* 85: 407, 1995

Cornell Bell A, Sullivan D, Allansmith M. Gender-related difference in the morphology of the lacrimal gland. *Invest Ophthal and Vis Sci.* 26:1170-1175,1985.

Cullberg J. Mood changes and menstrual symptoms with different gestagen/estrogen combinations. *Acta Psychiatr Scand (suppl)* 236: 1, 1972.

Cutler WB, Garcia CR, Huggins GR, et al. Sexual behavior and steroid levels among gynecologically premature premenopausal women. *Fertil Steril* 1986;48:496-502

Davis SR, McCloud P, Strauss BJG et al. Testosterone enhances estradiol's effects on postmenopausal bone density and sexuality. *Maturitas* 1995;21:227-36

Davis SR, Burger HG. Use of androgens in postmenopausal women. *Curr Opinion Obstet Gynecol* 9:177-80, 1997.

Davis SR. When to suspect androgen deficiency other than at menopause. *Fertil Steril* 2002; 77 [Suppl 4]: S68-S71.

Davison S,Bell R,Donath S,Montalto J,Davis S.Changes in androgen levels across the adult female life cycle. Abstract:The Endocrine Society Annual Meeting;June 16-19,2004;New Orleans,LA.

Decensi A, Omodei U, Robertson C, et al. Effect of transdermal estradiol and oral conjugated estrogen on C-reactive protein in retinoid-placebo trial in healthy women. *Circulation* 2002; 106:1224-1228.

Deeks AA,McCabe MP.Well-being and menopause:an investigation of purpose in life,self-acceptance and social role in premenopausal,perimenopausal and postmenopausal women.*Qual Life Res* .2004;13:389-398.

De Lignieres B, Dennerstein L, Backstrom T. Influence of route of administration on progesterone metabolism. *Maturitas* 21, 251-257, 1995

De Ziegler D, Meldrum DR. From in vitro fertlization (IVF) to menopause: physiologic hormone replacement adapted from donor egg IVF may be our best option for hormone therapy. *Fertil Steril* 2003; 80:485-487.

Dennerstein L, Dudley E, Burger H. Are changes in sexual functioning during midlife due to aging or menopause? *Fertil Steril* .2001;76:456-460.

Dennerstein L,Randolph J,Taffe J,Dudley E,Burger H. Hormones,mood, sexuality, and the menopausal transition. *Fertil Steril* .2002;77 suppl 4:S42-S48.

Dennerstein L, Randolph J, Taffe J, et al. Hormones, mood, sexuality, and the menopausal transition. *Fertil Steril* 2002;77:S42-S48

Deuschle M, Luppa P, Gilles M, et al. Antidepressant treatment and dehydro-epiandrosterone sulfate: different effects of amitriptyline and paroxetine. *Neuropsychobiology* 2004;50:252-256

Diamond, P., Cusan, L., Gomez, J.L. *et al.* (1996) Metabolic effects of 12-month percutaneous dehydroepiandrosterone replacement therapy in postmeno-pausal women. *J. Endocrinol.*, **150**, 543–550.

Dickey, R.P. Managing Contraceptive Pill Patients. Eleventh Edition, 2002. Available from: Essential Medical Information Systems, Inc., P.O. Box 820062, Dallas, TX 75382 or website: www.emispub.com

Dimitrakakis C, Zhou J, Bondy CA. Androgens and mammary growth and neoplasia. *Fertil Steril* 2002;77:S26-S33

Dionyssiou-Asteriou A, Drakakis P, Vatalas IA, Michalas S. Variations of serum hormone levels in young exercising women. *Clin Endocrinol* (Oxf). 51(2):258-260, 1999.

Dow MGT, Hart DM. Hormonal treatments of sexual unresponsiveness in postmeno-pausal women: a comparative study. *Br J Obstet Gynaecol* 1983; 90:361-6

Dunn KM, Croft PR, Hackett GI. Association of sexual problems with social, psychological, and physical problems in men and women: a cross sectional population survey. *J Epidemiol Community Health* 1999;53:144-148.

Eden JA. A pilot study of andro-feme cream (1%testosterone). In: Proceedings of the 4th Annual Congress of the Australasian Menopause Society; 2000; Adelaide, SA, Australia.

Everson RB, Sandler DR, Wilcox AJ, et al. Effect of passive exposure to smoking on age at natural menopause. *Br Med J* 293: 272, 1986

Floter A, Nathorst-Boos J, Carlstrom BK, et al. Androgen status and sexual life in perimenopausal women. *Menopause* 1997;4:95-100

Ferraroni Am, Dearli A, Franceschi S and La Vecchia C. Alcohol consumption and risk of breast cancer: a multicentre Italian case-control study. *European J of Cancer* 1998; 34:1403-1409.

Ferriman D, Gallwey JD. Clinical assessment of body hair growth in women with hyperandrogenism. *Endocrinol Metab* 1961;21:1440-47

Gambacciani M, Genazzani AR. Hormone therapy: the benefits in tailoring the regimen and dose. *Maturitas* 2001; 40:195-201.

Gambacciani M, Genazzani AR. The Missing R. (editorial). *Gynecol.Endocrinol* 2003; 17:91-94.

Gelfand M. Estrogen-androgen hormone replacement therapy. *European Menopause Journal* 2:22-26, 1995.

Genazzani AR, Gadducci A, Gambacciani M. Controversial issues in climacteric medicine II: Hormone replacement therapy and cancer. International Menopause Society Expert Position Paper. *Gynecol Endocrinol* 2001; 15:453-465.

Genazzani, AR (President of the International Menopause Society). HRT and breast cancer: is there any news? A clinician's perspective (editorial). *Climacteric: The Journal of the International Menopause Society*, 2000:3:13-16

Genazzani AR, Bernardi F, Spinetti A, et al. The brain as target and source for sex steroid hormones. Third International Symposium Women's Health and Menopause. June, 1998.

Genazzani AR, Gambacciani, M. A personal initiative for women's health: to challenge the Women's Health Initiative, *Gynecol Endocrinol* 16:255-257, August, 2002.

Goldstat R, Briganti, Tran J, et al. Transdermal testosterone therapy improves well-being, mood, and sexual function in premenopausal women. *Menopause* 2003; 10:390-8

Goldstat R, Briganti E, Tran J, et al. Transdermal testosterone therapy improves well-being, mood, and sexual function in premenopausal women. *Menopause* 2003;10:390-398

Gordon CM. Menstrual disorders in adolescents. Excess androgens and the polycystic ovary syndrome. *Pediatr Clin North Am.* 46(3):519-43,1999.

Govoni, S. Estrogens as neuroprotectants: Hypotheses on the mechanism of action. Third International Symposium Women's Health and Menopause, June, 1998

Gracia CR, Sammel MD, Freeman EW, et al. Predictors of decreased libido in women during the late reproductive years. *Menopause* 2004;11:144-150.

Graziottin A. Libido: the biologic scenario, *Maturitas* 2000;43(suppl 1):59-S16

Greenblatt RB. Androgenic therapy in women. *Endocrinology* 1942; 2:665-6

Greenblatt RB, Karpas, A. Hormone therapy for sexual dysfunction. *Postgraduate Medicine* 1983; 74:78-89

Greenblatt RB, Warfield WE, Garner JF, et al. Evaluation of estrogen, androgen, and estrogen-androgen combination and a placebo in the treatment of menopause. *J Clin Endocrinol Metab* 1950; 10:1547-48

Gregoire AJP, Kumar R, Everett B, Henderson A, Studd JWW. Transdermal oestrogen for treatment of severe postnatal depression, *Lancet* 347: 930-933, 1996.

Guay AT. Screening for androgen deficiency in women: methodological and interpretive issues. *Fertil Steril* 2002; 77: S83-S88

Hakkinen K, Pakarinen A. Acute hormonal changes to heavy resistance exercise in men and women at different ages. *Int. J. Sports Med.* 16(8), 507, 1995.

Haning, R.V. Jr., Hackett, R.J., Flood, C.A. *et al.* Plasma dehydroepiandrosterone sulfate serves as a prehormone for 48% of follicular fluid testosterone during treatment with menotropins. *J. Clin. Endocrinol. Metab.*1993; **76**, 1301–1307.

Harrison RL, Read GF. Ovarian impairments of female recreational distance runners during a season of training. *Annals of Human Biology* 25(4)345-357, 1998.

Hillen T, et al. DHEA-S plasma levels and incidence of Alzheimer's disease. *Biol Psychiatr* 2000; 47:161-163.

Hinson JP, Brooke A, Raven PW. Therapeutic uses of dehydroepiandrosterone. *Curr Opin Investig Drugs.* 2003;10:1205-8.

Hoek A, Schoemaker J, Drexhage HA. Premature ovarian failure and ovarian autoimmunity. *Endocrinology Review,* 18(1): 107-134, 1997.

Holst J, Backstrom T, Hammerbach S, et al. Progestogen addition during oestrogen replacement therapy – effects on vasomotor symptoms and mood. *Maturitas* 1989;11:13-19,

Hornsby PJ. Biosynthesis of DHEAS by the human adrenal cortex and its age-related decline. *Ann NY Acad Sci* 1995;774:29-46

Hunt PJ, Gurnell EM, Huppert FA, et al. Improvement in mood and fatigue after dehydroepiandrosterone treatment in Addison's disease in a randomized double-blind trial. *JCEM* 2000;85:4650-6

Jaussi R, Watson G, Paigen K. Modulation of androgen-responsive gene expression by estrogen, *Mol Cell Endocrinol.* 1992; 86:187.

Johannsson G, Burman P, Wiren L, et al. Low dose dehydroepiandrosterone affects behavior in hypopituitary androgen-deficient women: a placebo-controlled trial. *JCEM* 2002;87:2046-52

Joura EA, et al; Short-term effects of topical testosterone in vulvar lichen sclerosus.

Judd HL, Fournet N. Changes of ovarian hormonal function with aging. *Experiment Gerontol* 1994; 29:285-98

Judd HL, Lucas WE, Yen SS. Effect of oophrectomy on circulating testosterone and androstenedione levels in patients with endometrial cancer. *Am J. Obstet Gynecol* 1974;118:793-8

Kaplan HS. Disorders of sexual desire and other new concepts and techniques in sex therapy. Brunner/Mazel Publications, New York, NY, 1979.

Kaye, S.A., Folsom, A.R., Soler, J.T., Prineas, R.J. and Potter, J.D. Association of body mass and fat distribution with sex hormone concentrations in post-menopausal women. *Int. J. Epidemiol.*, 20, 151-6

Keizer H, Janssen GME, Menheere P, and Kranenburg G. Changes in basal plasma testosterone, cortisol, and dehydroepiandrosterone in previously untrained males and females preparing for a marathon. *Int. J. Sports Med.* 10, S139, 1989.

Khastgir G, Studd JWW. Hysterectomy, ovarian failure and depression. *Menopause* 5:113-122, 1998.

Kicman AT, Bassindale T, Cowan DA, et al. Effect of androstenedione ingestion on plasma testosterone in young women: a dietary supplement with potential health risks. *Clin Chem* 2003;49:167-9

Kim JG, Moon SY, Chang YS, Lee JY. Autoimmune ovarian failure. *Br J Obstet Gynaecol* 1995;21:59-66

Kingsberg SA. The impact of aging on sexual function in women and their partners. *Arch Sex Behav* 2002;31:431-437

Klaiber E, Broverman D, Vogel W, et al. Relationships of serum oestradiol levels, menopausal duration and mood during hormone replacement therapy. *Psychoneuroendocrinology* 22:549-58, 1997

Kolodny RC, Masters WH, Johnson VE. Textbook of Sexual Medicine. Little, Brown, Boston, 1979.

Kosta T, Patricot MC, Mathian B, et al Effects of exercise on estradiol levels in early postmenopausal women. *Aging Clin Exp Res.* 2003 Apr;15(2):123-30

Kyllonen ES, Vaananen HK, Heikkinen JE, et al. Comparison of Muscle strength and bone mineral density in healthy postmenopausal women: a cross-sectional population study. *Scand J Rehab Med* 23, 153-7, 1991.

Labrie F. Extragonadal synthesis of sex steroids: intracrinology . *Ann Endocrinol* 2003;64:95-107

Labrie F, Luu-The V, Lin SX, et al. Intracrinology: role of the family of 17B-hydroxysteroid dehydrogenases in human physiology and disease. *J Mol Endocrinol* 2000; 25:1-16

Labrie F, Luu-the V, Labrie C, et al. Endocrine and intracrine sources of androgens in women: inhibition of breast cancer and other roles of androgens and their precursor dehydroepiandrosterone. *Endoc Rev* 2003; 24: 152-82

Labrie F, Belanger A, Cusan L, et al. Marked decline in serum concentrations of adrenal C19 sex steroid precursors and conjugated androgen metabolites during aging. *JCEM* 1997;82:2396-2402

Lasley Bl, Santoro N, Randolf JF, et al. The relationship of circulating dehydro-epiandtrosterone, testosterone, and estradiol to stages of the menopausal transition and ethnicity. *JCEM* 2002; 87:3760-7

Laughlin GA, Barrett-Connor E, Kritz-Silverstein D, et al. Hysterectomy, oopho-rectomy and endogenous sex hormone levels in older women: the Rancho Bernardo Study. *J Clin Endocrinol Metab* 2000;85:645-51

Laumann EO, Paik A, Rosen RC. Sexual dysfunction in the United States: prevalence and predictors. *JAMA* 1999;281:537-544

Lebenstedt M., Platte P, Pirke KM. Reduced resting metabolic rate in athletes with menstrual disorders. *Med Sci Sports Exerc,* 31(9):1250-6, 1999.

Leder BZ, Leblanc KM, Longcope C, et al. Effects of oral androstenedione ad-ministration on serum testosterone and estradiol levels in postmenopausal women. *J Clin Endocrinol Metab* 2002;87:5449-54

Liu D, Dillon JS. Dehydroepiandrosterone activates endothelial cell nitric-oxide synthetase by a specific plasma membrane receptor couplet to $G\alpha_{12,}\alpha_{13.}$ *Biol Chem* 2002; 277:21379-21388.

Lobo RA, Rosen RC, Yang, HM, et al. Comparative effects of oral esterified estrogens with and without methyltestosterone on endocrine profiles and dimensions of sexual function in postmenopausal women with hypoactive sexual desire. *Fertil Steril* 2003; 79: 1341-52

Locke RJ, Warren MP. Exercise and primary dysmenorrhoea.*Br J Sports Med.* 33(4):227, 1999 Aug

Longcope C. Androgen Metabolism and the menopause. *Sem Reprod Endocrinol* 1998; 16:111-5

Longcope C. Adrenal and gonadal androgen secretion in normal females.*JCEM* 1986; 15:213-28

Longcope C, Hunter R, Franz C. Steroid secretion by the postmenopausal ovary. *Am J Obstet Gynecol* 1980; 1 38: 564-9

Longcope C, Franz C, Morello C, et al. Steroid and gonadotropin levels in women during the peri-menopausal years. *Maturitas* 1986;8:189-196

Longcope C. The male and female reproductive systems in hypothyroidism. In: *Werner and Ingbar's The Thyroid: Seventh Edition*, LE Braverman and RD Utiger (Eds), Lippincott-Raven, Philadelphia, 1996.

Mah K, Binik YM, The nature of human orgasm: a critical review of major trends. *Clin Psychol Rev* 2001;21:823-56

Masters WH, Johnson VE. Human Sexual Response. Little, Brown and Co., Boston, 1966

McClamrock H, Adashi E. Gestational Hyperandrogenism. *Fertil Steril* 1992;57:257-270

McCoy NL, Davidson JM. A longitudinal study of the effects of menopause on sexuality. *Maturitas* 1985;7:203-210

Mello N, Mendelson, J, Teoh S. Neuroendocrine Consequences of Alcohol Abuse in Women. *Ann NY Acad Sci* 1989; 562: 211-40

Metka M, Enzelsberger H, Knogler W, et al. Ophthalmic complaints as a climacteric symptom. *Maturitas* 14:3-8, 1991.

Miller KK, Sesmilo G, Schiller A, at al. Androgen deficiency in women with hypopituitarism. *J Clin Endocrinol Metab* 2001;86:51-7

Montgomery J, Brincat M, Appleby L, et al. Effect of oestrogen and testosterone implants on psychological disorders in the climacteric. *The Lancet* 1987;1:297-299

Morales AJ, Haubrich RH, Hwang JY, et al. The effect of six months treatment with a 100 mg daily dose of dehydropepiandrosterone (DHEA) on circulating sex steroids, body composition and muscle strength in age advanced men and women. *Clin Endocrinol* (Oxf) 1998;49:422-32

Morales AJ, Nolan JJ, Nelson JC, et al. Effects of replacement dose of dehydroepiandrosterone in men and women of advancing age. *J Clin Endocrinol Metab* 1994; 78:1360–1367.

Mortola JF, Yen SS. The effects of oral dehydroepiandrosterone on endocrine-metabolic parameters in postmenopausal women. *J Clin Endocrinol Metab* 1990; 71:1360-1367.

Morris NM, Udry JD, Khan-Dawood F, et al. Marital sexual frequency and midcycle female testosterone. *Arch Sex Behav* 1987;16:27-38

Muechler EK, Huang KE and Schenk E. Autoimmunity in premature ovarian failure. *International J Fertility* 36(2): 99-103, 1991.

Mushayandebvu T, Castracane DV, Gimpel T, et al. Evidence for diminished midcycle ovarian androgen production in older reproductive aged women. *Fertil Steril* 1996;65:721-723

Myers LS, Dixen J, Morrissette D, et al. Effects of estrogen, androgen, and progestin on sexual psychophysiology and behavior in postmenopausal women. *J Clin Endocrinol Metab* 1990;70:1124-31

Nieschlag E, Behre HM (Editors) <u>Testosterone: Action, Deficiency, Substitution, 2<u>nd</u> Edition</u>. Springer-Verlag, Berlin. 1998

Nilas L, Christensen C. The Pathophysiology of peri-and menopausal bone loss. *Br J Obstet Gynaecol* 96:580-585,1989.

Notelovitz M. Androgen effects on bone and muscle. *Fertil Steril* 2002;77:S34-S41

Notelovitz, M. Estrogen therapy and variable-resistance weight training increase bone mineral in surgically menopausal women. *J Bone Mineral Research* 6(6); 583-590, 1991.

O'Meara ES, Rossing MA, Daling JR, et al. Hormone replacement therapy after a diagnosis of breast cancer in relation to recurrence and mortality. *J Nat Cancer Inst* 2001; 93:754-762.

Orentreich N, Brind H, Rizer RL, et al. Age changes and sex differences in serum dehydroepiandrosterone sulfate concentrations through adulthood. *J Clin Endocrinol Metab* 1984; 59:551-5

Parasrampuria J, Schwartz K, Potesch R. Quality control of dehydroepiandrosterone dietary supplement products. *JAMA* 1998;280:1565

Parish E, Fletcher CD, Hart DM, et al. The effects of hormone implants on serum lipoproteins and steroid hormones in bilaterally oophorectomised women. *Acta Endocrinol* 1984; 106:116-20

Persky H, Lief AL, Strauss D, et al. Plasma testosterone levels and sexual behavior of couple. *Arch Sex Behav* 1987; 7:157-73

Persky H, Dreisbach L, Miller WR, et al. The relation of plasma androgen levels to sexual behaviors and attitudes of women. *Psychosom Med* 1982;44:305-19

Peterson HB et al. The risk of menstrual abnormalties after tubal sterilization. *N Engl J Med* 2000 Dec. 7; 343:1681-7

Phillip SK, Gopinathan J, Meehan K, Bruce S, and Woledge R. Muscle strength changes during the menstrual cycle in human adductor pollicis, *J. Physiol.* 473, 125P, 1993

Philllip SK, Rook K, Siddle N, Bruce S, and Woledge R. Muscle weakness in women occurs at an earlier age than in men, but strength is preserved by hormone replacement therapy. *Clin. Sci.* 84, 95, 1993.

Pirke KM, Schweiger U, Lemmel W, et al. The influence of dieting on the menstrual cycle of healthy young women. *J Clin Encdocrinology Metab* 60(6):1174-1179, 1985.

Pirke K, Schweiger U, Laessle R, et al. Dieting Influences the Menstrual Cycle: Vegetarian Versus Nonvegetarian Diet. *Fertility and Sterility* 1968; 46(6): 1083-1088

Raisz LG, Wiita B, Arjtis A, et al. Comparison of the effects of estrogen alone and estrogen plus androgen on biochemical markers of bone formation and resorption in postmenopausal women. *J Clin Endocrinol Metab* 1996;81:37-43

Rannevik G, Jeppsson S, Johnell O, et al. A longitudinal study of the perimenopausal transition: altered profiles of steroid and pituitary hormones, SHBG and bone mineral density. *Maturitas* 1995; 21:103-13

Redmond, GP. Androgenic Disorders, Raven Press, New York, 1995.

Rein, M., Jackson, K., Sable, D. *et al.* (1996) Dexamethasone during ovulation induction for in-vitro fertilization: a pilot study. *Hum. Reprod.*, **11**, 253–255.

Rossouw JE, Anderson GL, Prentice RL, et al. Risks and benefits of estrogen plus progestin in healthy postmenopausal women: principal results from the Women's Health Initiative randomized controlled trial. *JAMA* 2002;288:3231-333

Sarrel P, Dobay B, Wiita. Estrogen and estrogen-androgen replacement in postmenopausal women dissatisfied with estrogen only therapy. *J Reprod Med* 1998;43:847-56

Sarrel P. Effects of hysterectomy without oophorectomy on menopausal symptoms. Oral presentation, North American Menopause Society, New York, September 21-23, 1989.

Sarwar R, Beltran-Niclos B, and Rutherford O. Changes in muscle strength, relaxation rate, and fatiguability during the human menstrual cycle. *J. Physiol.* 493, 267, 1996.

Scarabin P, Oger E, Plu-Bureau G (for the EStrogen and THromboEmbolism Risk [ESTHER] Study Group. Differential association of oral and transdermal oestrogen replacement therapy with venous thromboembolism risk. *Lancet* 2003; 362:428-432.

Schneider, HPG. The view of the International Menopause Society on the women's health initiative (WHI). *Climacteric* 5:211-216, September, 2002.

Schneider, HPG. Guidelines for the hormone treatment of women in the menopausal transition and beyond. Position Statement by the Executive Committee of the

International Menopause Society. *Climacteric* 2004;7:8-11.

Schreiner-Engle P, Schiavi RC, Strum D, et al. Sexual arousability and the menstrual cycle. *Psychosom Med* 43:199, 1980.

Schreiner-Engle P, Schiavi RC, White D, et al. Low sexual desire in women: the role of reproductive hormones. *Horm Behav* 1989;23:221-34

Shangold M. Exercise and the Adult Female: Hormonal and Endocrine Effects. *Exer & Sport Sci Rev* 1984; 12: 53-79

Shaywitz SE, Shaywitz BA, Pugh KR, et al. Effect of estrogen on brain activation patterns in postmenopausal women during working memory tasks. *JAMA* 281(13):1197-1202, 1999.

Sherwin BB, Hormones, mood and cognitive functioning in postmenopausal women. *Obstet Gynecol* 87:20-26, 1996.

Sherwin BB, Gelfand MM. Differential symptom response to parenteral estrogen and/or androgen administration in surgical menopause. *Am J Obstet Gynecol*; 151: 153-158, 1985.

Sherwin BB, Tulandi T. 'Add-back' estrogen reverses cognitive deficits induced by a gonadotropin releasing-hormone agonist in women with leiomyomata uteri. *JCEM* 81:2545-2549, 1996.

Sherwin BB, Gelfand MM, Brender W. Androgen enhances sexual motivation in females: a prospective, crossover study of sexual steroid administration in surgical menopause. *Psychosom Med* 1985;47:339-51

Sherwin BB, Gelfand MM. Differential symptoms response to parenteral estrogen and/or androgen administration in the surgical menopause. *Am J. Obstet Gynecol* 1985;1512:153-9

Sherwin BB. Affective changes with oestrogen and androgen replacement therapy in surgically menopausal women. *J Affect Dis* 1988;14:177-87

Sherwin BB, Gelfand M. The role of androgen in the maintenance of sexual functioning in ovarectomized women. *Psychosom Med* 1987;49:397-409

Shifren JL, Braunstein GD, Simon JA, et al. Transdermal testosterone treatment in women with impaired sexual function after oopherectomy. *N Engl J Med* 2000;343:682-8

Simpson ER. Aromatization of androgens in women: current concepts and findings. *Fertil Steril* 2002; 77:S6-S10

Sinha-Hakim I, Arver S, Beall G, et al. The use of a sensitive equilibrium dialysis method for the measurement of five testosterone levels in healthy, cycling women and in human immunodeficiency virus-infected women. *J Clin Endocrinol Metab* 1998; 83:1312-1318

Smith RNJ, Studd JWW, Zamblera D, et al. A randomized comparison over 8 months of 100 mcgs and 200 mcgs twice weekly doses of transdermal oestradiol in the treatment of severe premenstrual syndrome. *Br J Obstet Gynaecol* 102: 475-484, 1995.

Somboonporn W, Davis SR. Testosterone effects on the breast: implications for testosterone therapy for women. *Endocrine Reviews* 2004; 25(3):374-388.

Speroff, L. Postmenopausal estrogen-progestin therapy and breast cancer: a clinical response to epidemiological reports. *Climacteric: The Journal of the International Menopause Society* 2000:3:3-12

Stickler RC. Women's health initiative results: a glass more empty than full. *Fertility and Sterility* 2003; 80:488-90.

Stott CA. Steroid hormones: metabolism and mechanism of action. *In* Yen SS, Jaffe RB, Barbieri RL (eds). <u>Reproductive Endocrinology: Physiology, Pathophysiology, and Clinical Management</u>. 4 ed. Philadelphia WB Saunders Co, 1999:124

Studd JWW, Collins WP, Chakravarti S, et al. Oestradiol and testosterone implants in the treatment of psychosexual problems in the postmenopausal woman. *Br J. Obstet Gynaecol* 1977; 84:314-5

Tarnopolsky M. <u>Gender Differences in Metabolism: Practical and Nutritional Implications</u>. CRC Press, New York and London, 1999.

Tchernof A, et al. Menopause, central body fatness, and insulin resistance: effects of hormone-replacement therapy. Coron Artery Dis. 9(8):503-11, 1998.

The Writing Group for the PEPI Trial. Effects of estrogen or estrogen/progestin regimens on heart disease risk factors in postmenopausal women: the postmenopausal estrogen/progestin intervention (PEPI) trial. JAMA 273:199-208, 1995.

The Writing Group for the Women's Health Initiative Investigators. Risks and benefits of estrogen plus progestin in healthy postmenopausal women. JAMA 2002;288:321-333.

Thijssen JHH, Nieuwenhuyse H (Editors). <u>DHEA: A Comprehensive Review</u>. The Parthenon Publishing Group, New York and London, 1999.

Tuiten A, VonHonk J, Koppeschaar H, et al. Time course of effects of testosterone administration on sexual arousal in women. *Arch Gen Psychiatry* 2000;57:149-53

VanGoozen SHM, Wiegant VM, Endert E, et al. Psychoendocrinological assessment of the menstrual cycle: the relationship between hormones, sexuality, and mood. *Arch Sex Behav* 1997;26:359-82

Van Vollenhoven RF, McGuire JL. Estrogen, progesterone and testosterone: can they be used to treat autoimmune diseases? *Cleve Clin J Med* 61: 276-284, 1994.

Valimaki N, Harkonen M, and Ylikahri R. Acute effects of alcohol on female sex hormones. *Alcohol Clin Exp Res* 7: 289-293, 1983. Vermeulen A. Plasma androgens in women. *J Reprod Med* 1998; 43: 725-33

VanThiel D, Lester R: The effects of chronic alcohol abuse on sexual function. JCEM 8:499, 1979

Vehkavaara S, Hakala-Ala-Pietila T, Virkamaki A, et al. Differential effects of oral and transdermal estrogen replacement therapy on endothelial function in postmenopausal women. *Circulation* 1999;102:2687-93

Vermeulen A, Verdonck L, Kaufman JM. A critical evaluation of simple methods for the estimation of free testosterone in serum. *J Clin Endocrinol Metab* 2999; 84:3666-72

Vermeulen A, Verdonck L. Plasma androgen levels during the menstrual cycle. *Am J. Obstet Gynecol* 1976;125:491-4

Vintamaki T, Tuimala R. Can climacteric women self-adjust therapeutic estrogen doses using symptoms as markers? *Maturitas*, 1998; 199-203.

Vliet, EL An approach to perimenopausal migraine. *Menopause Management*, 4(6): 25-33, 1995.

Vliet, EL. Hormone connections in urinary incontinence in women. *Top Ger Rehab*; 15(4):16-30, 2000.

Vliet, EL. It's My Ovaries, Stupid! Scribner, New York, 2003,

Vliet EL. Menopause and perimenopause: role of ovarian hormones in common neuroendocrine syndromes in primary care. Primary Care Clinics in Office Practice, 2002, 29:43-67.

Vliet EL, Davis VL New perspectives on the relationship of hormonal changes to affective disorders in the perimenopause. In Clinical Issues in Women's Health, Vol. 2, (4): Midlife Women's Health, Oct-Dec, JB Lippincott, Philadelphia, 1991, pp 453-472.

Vliet, EL. Screaming to Be Heard: Hormone Connections Women Suspect and Doctors Still Ignore. (Revised edition) M. Evans and Company, New York, 2001.

Vliet, EL. Women, Weight and Hormones. M. Evans and Company, New York, 2001.

Watson NR, Studd JWW, Garnett T, et al. Bone loss after hysterectomy with ovarian conservation. Ostet Gynecol 86(1): 72-77,1995.

Watts NB, Notelovitz M, Timmons MC, et al. Comparison of oral estrogens and estrogens plus androgen on bone mineral density, menopausal symptoms, and lipid-lipoprotein profiles in surgical menopause. Obstet Gynecol. 85:529-537, 1995.

Wheatcroft NJ, Rogers CA, Metcalfe RA, et al., Is subclinical ovarian failure an autoimmune disease? Human Reproduction 12:244-249, 1997.

Whitehead, M. Oestrogens: relative potencies and hepatic effects after different routes of administration J Obstet Gynecology 3(suppl) S11-16,1982.

Whitehead M. (Ed.) The Prescriber's Guide to Hormone Replacement Therapy. Parthenon Publishing Group, New York and London, 1998.

Whitten PL, Lewis C, Russell E, Naftolin F. Potential adverse effects of phytoestrogens. Journal of Nutrition 125(Suppl):S 776, 1995.

Williams M, Ling S, Dawood T, et al. Dehydroepiandrosterone inhibits human vascular smooth muscle cell proliferation independent of ARs and ERs. J Clin Endocrinol Metab 2002; 87:176-181.

Williams NI, Bullen BA, McArthur JW, et al. Effects of short–term strenuous exercise upon corpus luteum function. Med Sci Sports Exerc 31(7):949-958, 1999.

Worboys S, Kotsopoulos D, Teede H, et al. Parental testosterone improves endothelium-dependent and independent vasodilation in postmenopausal women already receiving estrogen. J Clin Endocrinal Metab 2001;86:158-161

Wren BG, McFarland K, Edwards P, et al. Effect of sequential transdermal progesterone cream on endometrium, bleeding pattern, and plasma progesterone and salivary progesterone levels in postmenopausal women. Climacteric 2000;3:155-160

Yen SS. Effects of lifestyle and body composition on the ovary (review). Endocrinol Metab Clin North Am.27(4):915-926,1998.

Zhou J, Ng S, Andesanya-Famuiya O, et al. Testosterone inhibits estrogen-induced mammary epithelial proliferation and suppresses estrogen receptor expression. FASEB J 2000;14:1725-30

Zumoff B, Strain GW, Miller LK, et al. Twenty-four hour mean plasma testosterone concentration declines with age in normal premenopausal women. J Clin Endocrinol Metab 1995;80:1329-30

II. Groups and Organizations

American Association of Sex Educators, Counselors, and Therapists. www.aasect.org. If you are looking for a therapist who specializes in sexual problems, this is a good organization to check for licensed professionals in your area.

International Society for the Study of Androgen Insufficiency (formerly, The Andropause Society). www.andropause.org.uk. This organization specifically focuses on international research and clinical approaches for men and women with androgen deficiency. Their website has abstracts from recent conferences on the effects of androgens in men and women.

International Menopause Society, www.imsociety.org. This organization is an international group of health professionals involved in basic and clinical research and patient care for women (and men) in the climacteric and menopausal years. The IMS publishes *Climacteric*, one of the leading medical journals devoted to cutting edge research from around the world in this field. The editors have refused to take advertising for products that have not been proven effective in properly designed, controlled clinical trials. In my opinion, it is the best available for a balanced, non-commercial resource, presenting studies of hormone effects on brain and body, as well as comparison studies of different types of hormone preparations.

International Society of Gynecological Endocrinology. www.gynecologicalendocrinology.org. The professional organization for physicians and health professionals worldwide who specialize in the evaluation and treatment of various gynecologic endocrine disorders, from precocious puberty to infertility to menopause. Their journal, *Gynecological Endocrinology*, is an excellent and very broad-based resource for articles on research being conducted world-wide in this field.

National Osteoporosis Foundation (NOF), www.nof.org. An excellent source of cutting edge information about osteoporosis prevention and treatment. Join NOF and become an advocate in your community. I highly recommend their educational materials

PolyCystic Ovarian Syndrome Association, Inc. www.pcosupport.com. An excellent resource for educational materials, support groups, web discussions of PCOS. The organization also hosts an outstanding annual conference on PCOS, with presentations from many of the leading experts in the field. Check out their Web site at, or call 630-585-3690. Mail address is P.O. Box 7007, Rosemont, IL 60018

Sexuality Information and Education Council of the U.S. www.siecus.org. One of the organizations that pioneered the study of human sexuality. There are many reputable resources available through this group.

Sources For Natural Hormones

Disclaimer: *I have no financial interest in any of these pharmacies or their products.* I provide this information as a service to you and your physician because reliable information on these topics has been difficult for the average consumer to obtain. Compounded and "natural" hormones are not new, in spite of all the recent marketing of such products. Many of these options have been around for forty years or more. I have been a longstanding advocate for the use of bio-identical, "natural" human forms of hormone preparations, and I have seen over many years of my practice the marked positive difference that occurs when women change from the animal-derived, conjugated estrogens and synthetic forms of progestins.

Belmar Pharmacy, Charles Hakala, R.Ph., Lakewood, CO (Denver area)
    Phone 800-525-9473 Fax 303-763-9712

Charles Hakala has been a pioneer in compounding prescriptions for patients with challenging medical problems such as chemical sensitivities, multiple allergies to dyes/binders, in addition to his outstanding reputation in the field of compounding natural, bio-identical hormone preparations for thyroid, ovary, and adrenal hormones. Charles is also knowledgeable about important differences between the more reliable *serum* methods of hormone testing versus methods such as saliva and urine that commonly give misleading results. He will discuss these issues with both consumers and physicians. He uses micronized natural forms of estradiol, testosterone, progesterone, and DHEA derived from soybeans and wild yams, and will make prescriptions in whatever form is needed for best results. Belmar pharmacists will make up prescriptions using lactose-free hypoallergenic formulations with no dyes; they also make vaginal creams that are hypoallergenic and omit some of the common irritants found in most commercial products.

Spence Pharmacy, Daryl Spence, R.Ph., Ft. Worth, TX (Dallas-Ft. Worth Metroplex)
    Phone 800-209-7364 Fax 817-625-8103

Daryl Spence is another reliable compounding pharmacist who has created innovative topical pain relief medications, in addition to his work with bio-identical, natural micronized hormones such as estradiol, testosterone, progesterone, DHEA. Spence Pharmacy will also make up prescriptions using lactose-free hypoallergenic formulations with no dyes, and no preservatives that are potentially irritating or may aggravate allergies.

Both Belmar and Spence Pharmacies are *full-service pharmacies* with ability to fill all of your prescription needs, not just compounded prescriptions. In addition, I have found that both of these pharmacies often have better prices on common commercial prescriptions (suchas estradiol patches) than my patients find at the big chain drugstores. I encourage you to do a little price-shopping to decide where you want your prescriptions filled before you automatically assume the big chain drugstores are cheaper.

General Comments about Compounded Hormones

There are many pharmacies around the country that are now providing compounding services. There are several important reasons I have continued to collaborate primarily with Belmar and Spence pharmacies on prescriptions for my patients.

First, both of these pharmacists have many years' experience in the art and science of compounding and are not just starting these services in the wake of current interest. Neither pharmacy is "selling" hormone consults based on saliva tests. They will work with patients and physicians to determine appropriate options.

Second, each compounding pharmacist has his or her own formula for making the various forms of prescription hormones, and each formulation will vary in how it is metabolized in the body. Therefore, each formulation will act somewhat differently in a given person and adds yet another variable to the equation of trying to solve the problem when a person has side effects. It is difficult enough clinically to sort out individual differences in metabolism and response when I know the pharmacology of a given preparation. If the preparation also varies, it can become almost impossible to sort out the Gordian knot of factors that could alter a person's response.

That's why I prefer to work with brand name products instead of generics, and to limit my prescriptions to just a few compounding pharmacists upon whose preparations I can rely for consistency.

Third, I am increasingly concerned at the degree to which some pharmacists are now practicing medicine by adjusting women's hormone doses based on questionable test methods, such as saliva and urine hormone levels, without having access to other laboratory measures that need to be included in decision making about appropriate hormone dose and route. Pharmacists are not licensed to determine the *dose* that is correct for you; that function is by law the task of the physician. I have treated too many patients who have been significantly overdosed on hormones when getting their information from pharmacists making dose decisions and changes. I have chosen to only put my prescriptions at pharmacies where the pharmacists do not engage in this practice.

The two pharmacies I listed above are resources I have depended upon to provide individual prescriptions for my patients and family; we have been pleased with the results. These pharmacists are skilled, knowledgeable, and committed to providing quality service to you and your physician. I have found them to be ethical and responsible in working *with* the physician. Neither of these pharmacy owners allows their staff to go outside the bounds of pharmacy licensing and make dose decisions or changes on their own without consultation with your physician.

Compounded Hormones vs. FDA-Approved Hormones:

Women often ask, "Are these compounded hormones FDA-approved?" The answer is no, because the individual compounded prescriptions are not manufactured and distributed for sale in quantities that would require FDA-approval. At reputable compounding pharmacies, the ingredients used are *pharmaceutical-grade* (U.S.P.) bases that are then made up into tablets or creams or suppositories to your individual needs. Individual pharmacists operate within their training and state licenses when they prepare (compound) individual prescriptions based on your own physician's decision about dose and type of medication best for you.

FDA-approved hormone products are manufactured by major pharmaceutical companies for commercial distribution throughout the country. There are many FDA-approved *bioidentical* hormone products available today, so you do not have to use a compounding pharmacy to get bioidentical hormones. Most are covered on major health plan prescription programs.

Much of the current use of individual compounding is for patients with allergies, marked sensitivities to dyes and binders in commercial preparations, patients who need smaller doses, and in particular, women who want to take bioidentical testosterone, which is not yet available in an FDA-approved commercial product. **Do not try to use the men's testosterone patch or gel—the dose is far too high for women.**

To Contact Dr. Vliet

For Individual Medical Consultations:

1. We have a centralized appointment scheduling process for our consultations managed from the Tucson office.

   Please contact the Patient Services Coordinator in Tucson at *HER Place®: Health, Enhancement and Renewal for Women, Inc.* To receive an information package, you may mail request to P.O. Box 64507, Tucson, AZ 85728, or call 520-797-9131, Fax 520-797-2948.

2. You may check our website at www.herplace.com. Read about our services on the website, and you may also request to be added to our email "alert" notification list to receive periodic health notices. Then contact the Tucson office as shown above. Legal issues and state regulations prevent us from answering medical questions via the web. All new patients are seen in person for a comprehensive evaluation at one of our offices.

For Medical Professionals and Organizations:

To arrange SPEAKING ENGAGEMENTS, SEMINARS, or WORKSHOPS by Dr. Vliet, or a discuss PRECEPTORSHIP or Consulting Services FOR HEALTH PROFESSIONALS, please contact:

> Kathryn A. Kresnik
> Vice President, Business Development
> *HER Place®*
> Phone: 520-797-9131, Fax 520-797-2948.
> Email: via our website www.herplace.com
> Regular Mail: Use Tucson office address above